Clinical Examination Skills

The *Essential Clinical Skills for Nurses* series focuses on key clinical skills for nurses and other health professionals. These concise, accessible books assume no prior knowledge and focus on core clinical skills, clearly presenting common clinical procedures and their rationale, together with the essential background theory. Their user-friendly format makes them an indispensable guide to clinical practice for all nurses, especially to student nurses and newly qualified staff.

Other titles in the *Essential Clinical Skills for Nurses* series:

Central Venous Access Devices
Lisa Dougherty
ISBN: 9781405119528

Clinical Assessment and Monitoring in Children
Diana Fergusson
ISBN: 9781405133388

Intravenous Therapy
Theresa Finlay
ISBN: 9780632064519

Respiratory Care
Caia Francis
ISBN: 9781405117173

Care of the Neurological Patient
Helen Iggulden
ISBN: 9781405117166

ECGs for Nurses
Philip Jevon
ISBN: 9780632058020

Monitoring the Critically Ill Patient
Second Edition
Philip Jevon and Beverley Ewens
ISBN: 9781405144407

Treating the Critically Ill Patient
Philip Jevon
ISBN: 9781405141727

Pain Management
Eileen Mann and Eloise Carr
ISBN: 9781405130714

Leg Ulcer Management
Christine Moffatt, Ruth Martin and Rachael Smithdale
ISBN: 9781405134767

Practical Resuscitation
Edited by Pam Moule and John Albarran
ISBN: 9781405116688

Pressure Area Care
Edited by Karen Ousey
ISBN: 9781405112253

Infection Prevention and Control
Christine Perry
ISBN: 9781405140386

Stoma Care
Theresa Porrett and Anthony McGrath
ISBN: 9781405114073

Caring for the Perioperative Patient
Paul Wicker and Joy O'Neill
ISBN: 9781405128025

Clinical Examination Skills

Philip Jevon
RGN, BSc (Hon), PGCE, ENB 124
Resuscitation Officer/Clinical Skills Lead
Honorary Clinical Lecturer
Manor Hospital
Walsall
UK

With
Dr Gareth Walters
MB ChB BSc(Hons.) MRCP(UK) LCGI AHEA MInstLM
Specialist Registrar in Respiratory and
General Internal Medicine
West Midlands Rotation
Honorary Clinical Lecturer, University of Birmingham
UK

Dr Yi-Yang Ng
MBChB (Aberdeen) MRCS (UK)
ST trainee in General Practice, KSS Deanery
Honorary Clinical Lecturer, University of Birmingham
UK

Consulting Editor
Dr Alan Cunnington
BSc, MD, FRCP
Consultant Physician and Cardiologyist (Retired)
Manor Hospital, Walsall
UK

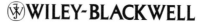
A John Wiley & Sons, Ltd., Publication

This edition first published 2009
© 2009 Philip Jevon

Blackwell Publishing was acquired by John Wiley & Sons in February 2007.
Blackwell's publishing programme has been merged with Wiley's global
Scientific, Technical, and Medical business to form Wiley-Blackwell.

Registered office
John Wiley & Sons Ltd, The Atrium, Southern Gate, Chichester, West Sussex,
PO19 8SQ, United Kingdom

Editorial offices
9600 Garsington Road, Oxford, OX4 2DQ, United Kingdom
2121 State Avenue, Ames, Iowa 50014-8300, USA

For details of our global editorial offices, for customer services and for information about how to apply for permission to reuse the copyright material in
this book please see our website at www.wiley.com/wiley-blackwell.

The right of the author to be identified as the author of this work has been
asserted in accordance with the Copyright, Designs and Patents Act 1988.

Wiley also publishes its books in a variety of electronic formats. Some
content that appears in print may not be available in electronic books.

Designations used by companies to distinguish their products are often
claimed as trademarks. All brand names and product names used in this
book are trade names, service marks, trademarks or registered trademarks of
their respective owners. The publisher is not associated with any product or
vendor mentioned in this book. This publication is designed to provide
accurate and authoritative information in regard to the subject matter
covered. It is sold on the understanding that the publisher is not engaged in
rendering professional services. If professional advice or other expert assis-
tance is required, the services of a competent professional should be sought.

Library of Congress Cataloging-in-Publication Data

Jevon, Philip.
   Clinical examination skills / Philip Jevon.
     p. ; cm. – (Essential clinical skills for nurses)
   Includes bibliographical references and index.
   ISBN 978-1-4051-7886-0 (pbk. : alk. paper)   1. Nursing assessment–
Handbooks, manuals, etc.   2. Medical history taking–Handbooks, manuals,
                        etc. I. title, II. Series.
   [DNLM: 1. Nursing Assessment–methods–Handbooks.   2. Medical
     History Taking–methods–Handbooks.   3. Physical Examination–
                   methods–Handbooks. WY 49 J86c 2008]
                           RT48.J48 2008
                           616.07′5–dc22
                               2008022317

A catalogue record for this book is available from the British Library.

Set in Set in 9 on 12 pt Palatino by SNP Best-set Typesetter Ltd., Hong Kong
Printed and bound in Malaysia by Vivar Printing Sdn Bhd.

1   2009

Contents

Foreword

Clinical examination has always been a cornerstone of nursing practice, and the development of examination skills is a crucial part of nurses' professional development. Examination skills enable nurses to monitor their patients and know when and how to act if there are causes for concern.

In the past, the majority of examinations undertaken by nurses would have been part of the ongoing monitoring and assessment performed between examinations undertaken by doctors. Although this is often still the case, nurses are taking a lead on patient care in a growing range of situations, and may be the only healthcare professional examining a particular patient. Even when they are working as part of a multidisciplinary team, nurses are often the only professionals in a position to see changes in a patient's condition at an early stage when intervention can avert a crisis.

Whatever the circumstances, it is vital that nurses undertake clinical examinations competently and thoroughly, and that they understand the implications of their results. This book will be an invaluable aid to this – both for nurses who are developing these skills for the first time and for those who want to refresh them and ensure that they are maintaining their competency. It offers a thorough exploration of all aspects of each examination, giving a clear rationale for undertaking it, putting symptoms in context and explaining the significance of the results. The different bodily systems and their examination are discussed separately, enabling readers to focus on each in turn, but the importance of combining them into a single, rounded intervention is emphasized. Learning outcomes for each chapter mean readers can test themselves to ensure that they have grasped the essentials, while the clear and logical format makes the book an ideal reference resource to return to for quick reminders.

Some examination procedures are often seen as 'routine' or 'basic' care to be delegated to the most junior member of the team. This misses the point. Although the individual practical procedures may be easily developed, it requires rather more to learn how to undertake a full clinical examination thoroughly, efficiently and sensitively – and to understand the implications of the results. It is refreshing, therefore, to see that the discussion is not restricted to practical skills. Readers are reminded to take a holistic approach, using communication skills and developing rapport in order to understand the patient's personal circumstances and how these might influence their condition. This often involves a certain amount of detective work, looking for clues to direct history taking and ongoing assessment along what might not be the most obvious route. Therefore, although it may be appropriate for junior staff to take on a certain amount of monitoring and assessment, we must not lose sight of the importance of having the input of an experienced practitioner at frequent intervals.

We hope that this book will help nurses to develop or refresh their examination skills and also to appreciate the importance of these skills and to see beyond the apparent simplicity of many individual elements of a clinical examination. A well-conducted examination may look straightforward, but it is the synthesis of a sophisticated array of skills and knowledge, as this valuable text clearly demonstrates.

Ann Shuttleworth and Kathryn Godfrey
Clinical Editors
Nursing Times

Preface

When I undertook my student nurse training in 1983–6, clinical examination was the realm of doctors. However, healthcare delivery is changing. With the emergence of nurse-led clinics, nurse-led minor injury units, walk-in centres, hospital-at-night services, etc., more and more nurses are now being required to perform some or all aspects of clinical examination. This trend is set to continue following the implementation of the European Union's Working Hour Directives and the reduction of junior doctors' working hours. Aspects of clinical examination skills are now included in pre-registration nursing curriculums.

'Clinical Examination Skills' is a new book written specifically for nurses. Providing an introduction to clinical examination (and history taking) skills, the book follows a methodical approach, describing each of the major bodily systems in turn. Although described separately in different chapters, the examination routines for each system should not be considered as entirely separate entities: when examining several systems at once, a single fluid routine should be used throughout the clinical examination; this will come with practice.

When undertaking clinical examination, the nurse must respect the patient as an individual, obtain consent and protect confidential information provided by the patient; in addition, the nurse should ensure that professional knowledge and competence in examination skills are maintained (Nursing and Midwifery Council, 2008).

It must be stressed that a different approach is advocated if the patient is critically ill; Chapter 8 outlines the ABCDE approach to assessment in this possibly life-threatening situation.

Philip Jevon

REFERENCE

Nursing and Midwifery Council (NMC) (2008) *The Code: Standards of Conduct, Performance and Ethics for Nurses and Midwives*. NMC, London.

Acknowledgements

I am grateful to Alan Cunnington for kindly checking the factual content of the book. I am also grateful to Gareth Walters and Yang Ng for contributing their chapters to the book.

I would like to thank Yang Ng (Clinical Advisor), Steve Webb (Photographer), Shareen Juwle (Nurse) and Joseph Seager (patient) for their help with the photographs.

Some of the text in chapter 3 may be similar to text in *Cardio-vascular examination parts 1–4 (vol 103: no 26, p28–29, no 27 p 26–27, no 28 p24–25, no 29 p26–27 (2007)*, articles I wrote with Dr Alan Cunnington, which were published in Nursing Times. I am grateful to EMAP for kindly granting me permission to reproduce text from these articles.

I am grateful to Ann Shuttleworth and Kathryn Godfrey, Clinical Editors at Nursing Times, for kindly writing the Foreword for the book.

Finally, I would like to thank Magenta Lampson and her colleagues at Wiley-Blackwell Publishing for their help, support and patience.

Philip Jevon

Overview of History Taking and Clinical Examination | **1**

INTRODUCTION

History taking (discussing patients' complaints with them) and clinical examination, together with performing or ordering relevant investigations, are important when trying to establish a diagnosis (Cox & Roper, 2005). Despite the advances in modern diagnostic tests, history taking and clinical examination remain fundamental to determining the most appropriate treatment (if any) for patients.

History taking and clinical examination require a structured, logical approach to ensure that all the relevant information is obtained and that nothing important is overlooked. History taking and clinical examination skills are difficult to acquire and, above all, require practice (Gleadle, 2004).

The aim of this chapter is to provide an understanding of the principles of history taking and clinical examination.

LEARNING OUTCOMES

At the end of this chapter, the reader will be able to:

❏ Discuss the objectives of history taking.
❏ Outline how to establish a rapport with the patient.
❏ Discuss the sequence of history taking.
❏ Discuss the symptoms of disease.
❏ Provide an overview to clinical examination.
❏ Outline the role of tests and investigations.

OBJECTIVES OF HISTORY TAKING

History taking is important for making a provisional diagnosis; clinical examination and investigations can then help to confirm or refute it. The history will provide information about the illness as well as the disease; the illness is the subjective component and describes the patient's experience of the disease (Shah, 2005a). A carefully taken medical history will provide the diagnosis or diagnostic possibilities in 78% of patients (Stride & Scally, 2005).

The objectives of history taking are to:

- Establish a rapport with the patient.
- Elicit the patient's presenting symptoms.
- Identify signs of disease.
- Make a diagnosis or differential diagnosis.
- Place the diagnosis in the context of the patient's life.

HOW TO ESTABLISH A RAPPORT WITH THE PATIENT

Establishing a rapport with the patient is essential. If patients believe that they are getting the nurse's full attention, they are more likely to try to accurately answer questions and recall past events.

To establish a rapport and to put the patient at ease, it is helpful to start the examination/interview by considering such issues as:

- *Positive initial contact*: shake the patient's hand whilst introducing yourself.
- *Privacy*: reassure patients that their privacy and dignity will be maintained.
- *Patient's name*: establish how the patient would like to be addressed (forename or surname).
- *Patient's physical comfort*: ensure that the patient is in a comfortable position and position yourself so that the patient is not sitting at an awkward angle.
- *Confidentiality*: reassure patients that all of their information will be treated as confidential.
- *Posture*: avoid standing up, towering over the patient; ideally sit down at the same level as the patient (Figure 1.1).
- *Effective communication skills* (Box 1.1): in particular, allow time to listen to what the patient is saying and avoid appearing to be rushed.

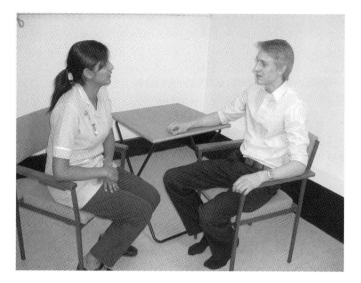

Fig 1.1 Helping to establish a rapport with the patient: sit down at the same level

---

Box 1.1 Effective communication skills required for history taking

History taking involves effective communication skills such as:

- Opening and closing a consultation.
- Using open and closed questions.
- Using non-verbal language.
- Active listening.
- Showing respect and courtesy.
- Showing empathy.
- Being culturally sensitive.

(Shah, 2005a)

- *Appropriate language*: appropriate language and understanding are important aspects of history taking; as the patient may not understand a particular word or phrase, always have an alternative available, e.g. 'sputum' or 'phlegm'; ensure that the patient understands the question or any information given (Shah, 2005b). Also, if the patient does not understand English, if possible communicate through an interpreter.

SEQUENCE OF HISTORY TAKING

The following sequence of history taking is recommended:

- Introduction.
- Presenting complaint and history of current illness.
- Systemic enquiry.
- Past medical history.
- Drugs.
- Allergies.
- Family history.
- Social and personal history.
- Patients' ideas, concerns and expectations.

(Source: Ford *et al.*, 2005)

Introduction

It is important to introduce yourself to the patient, e.g. name, position. Confirm the identity of patients: ask their name and how they prefer to be addressed. Consent should then be sought for history taking and clinical examination.

Presenting complaint and history of current illness

By far the most important part of history taking and clinical examination is the history of the patient's presenting complaint and history of current illness; the information elicited usually helps to make a differential diagnosis and provides a vital insight into the features of the complaints that the patient is particularly concerned about (Gleadle, 2004).

Therefore, a large part of history taking involves asking questions concerning the patient's presenting complaint(s) to establish the main symptom(s). The objective is to obtain a chronological account of the relevant events, including any interventions and outcomes, together with a detailed description of the patient's main symptoms (Ford *et al.*, 2005).

Ask patients to describe what has happened to bring them to hospital or to seek medical help. Their narrative will provide important clues as to the diagnosis and their perspective of the illness. Allow patients ample time to do this and it is important not to interrupt. Short responses, such as 'please tell me more', 'go on', etc., will encourage patients to elaborate.

Once the presenting complaint has been established, it must be carefully evaluated in detail:

- Start date/time.
- Who noticed the problem (patient, relative, caregiver, health-care professional)?
- What initial action did the patient take (any self-treatment) – did it help?
- When was medical help sought and why?
- What action was taken by the healthcare professional?
- What has happened since then?
- What investigations have been undertaken and what are planned?
- What treatment has been given?
- What has the patient been told about the problem?

(Source: Shah, 2005a)

Systemic enquiry

The systemic enquiry is a series of questions related to the bodily systems, which allows more information to be obtained that can be linked to the presenting complaint; considered as a safety net, it reduces the risk of missing an important symptom or disease (Shah, 2005b).

However, the systemic enquiry can cause confusion and mis-direct the clinician if the patient has multiple symptoms or is talkative or garrulous. It should therefore be undertaken system-atically and carefully: a suggested 'checklist approach' is detailed in Box 1.2.

It is standard practice to start with the most relevant system(s) to the presenting complaint. For example, if the patient pre-sents with chest pain, questions about the cardiovascular and

Box 1.2 Systemic enquiry

General:

- Well/unwell.
- Weight gain or loss.
- Appetite good or poor.
- Fevers.
- Sweats.
- Rigors.

Cardiovascular:

- Chest pain.
- Breathlessness.
- Orthopnoea.
- Paroxysmal nocturnal dyspnoea.
- Ankle swelling.
- Palpitations.
- Collapse.
- Exercise tolerance.
- Syncope.

Respiratory:

- Shortness of breath.
- Haemoptysis.
- Cough.
- Sputum.
- Wheeze.
- Pleuritic pain.

Nervous system:

- Headaches.
- Fits.
- Blackouts.
- Collapses.
- Falls.
- Weakness.
- Unsteadiness.
- Tremor.
- Visual and sensory disorders.
- Hearing disorder.

Gastrointestinal:

- Nausea.
- Vomiting.
- Diarrhoea.
- Abdominal pain.
- Mass.
- Rectal bleeding.
- Change in bowel habit.
- Dysphagia.
- Heartburn.
- Jaundice.
- Anorexia/weight loss.

Musculoskeletal:

- Weakness.
- Joint stiffness.
- Joint pain/swelling.
- Hot/red joints.
- Reduced mobility.
- Loss of function.

Genitourinary:

- Dysuria/urgency.
- Haematuria.
- Frequency.
- Nocturia.
- Urinary incontinence.
- Urethral/vaginal discharge.
- Menstrual cycle.
- Sexual function.

Skin:

- Rash.
- Lumps.
- Itching.
- Bruising.

respiratory systems should initially be asked (Shah, 2005b). The depth of questioning will depend on personal experience, the individual patient, the presenting complaint, the situation and circumstances.

Past medical history

It is useful to establish the patient's past medical history because:

- If the patient has a long-standing disease, there is a strong possibility that any new symptom could relate to it.
- It could help with making the correct diagnosis.
- It is helpful when establishing the most appropriate treatment for the patient.

Ask patients if they have ever had any serious illness, been admitted to hospital previously or had surgery. It is usual practice to record whether they have suffered from/suffer from any of the following illnesses:

- Jaundice.
- Anaemia.
- Tuberculosis.
- Rheumatic fever.
- Diabetes.
- Bronchitis.
- Myocardial infarction/chest pain.
- Stroke.
- Epilepsy.
- Asthma.
- Problems with anaesthesia.

(Gleadle, 2004)

Drugs

Obtaining a drug history is helpful because:

- Side-effects of drug therapy could be the cause of the patient's presenting complaint.
- Before starting or adjusting drug treatment, it is important to be aware of what the patient is already taking, e.g. old drug therapy could be ineffective or may interact with new drug therapy.

Establish if the patient is taking any of the following:

- Prescription drugs.
- Over-the-counter drugs, i.e. drugs bought without a prescription, e.g. aspirin.
- Herbal or 'natural' treatments.
- Illegal or recreational drugs.

(Shah, 2005b)

If the patient is taking medications, establish the dose, route of administration, frequency and duration of treatment. The possibility of non-compliance with prescription drugs should also be considered.

Patients may be unsure about what drugs they are taking. Under these circumstances, it is worthwhile using the medical history and asking them if they are taking any treatment for each problem, e.g. 'do you take anything for your arthritis?' (Shah, 2005b).

In addition, if patients know what drugs they are taking, it can be helpful to ask them what they are taking them for, because this may sometimes provide helpful additional information related to their illnesses (Shah, 2005b).

Allergies
An accurate and detailed description of any allergic responses of the patient to drugs or other allergens should be recorded; in particular, the patient should be asked about allergy to penicillin. If the patient has an allergy, try to determine what actually happened in order to differentiate between an allergy and a side-effect (Shah, 2005b): a side-effect refers to an effect of a drug which is not that which the doctor and patient require, whereas an allergy is a term usually used to describe an adverse reaction by the body to a substance to which it has been exposed (Marcovitch, 2005). The wearing of a 'medic alert' bracelet or similar (Figure 1.2) and the reason for doing so should be noted.

Family history
It is important to establish the diseases that have affected the patient's relatives, because there is a strong genetic contribution to many diseases (Gleadle, 2004).

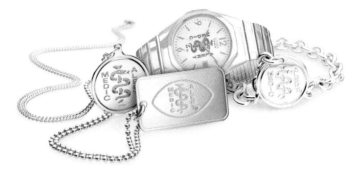

Fig 1.2 Medic alert devices (image supplied by Medic Alert, reproduced with permission)

Shah (2005b) recommends the following approach to taking a family history:

- Ascertain who has the problem: is it a first- or second-degree relative?
- Determine how many family members are affected by the problem.
- Clarify what exactly is the problem. For example, 'a problem with the heart' could be several things – hypertension, ischaemia, valve problems, etc. Be exact as to the nature of the problem, because several family members may have 'heart problems', but they may be completely different and therefore not relevant to the patient's particular problem.
- Determine at what age the relative developed the problem; obviously, early presentation is more likely to be important than presentation later in life.
- Ascertain if the patient's parents are still alive and, if not, at what age they died and the cause of death.

Social and personal history
Social history
It is important to understand the social history of patients: their background, the effect of their illness on their life and on the life of their family (Gleadle, 2004):

- *Marital status and children*: ask if they are married/have a partner and whether they have children. This is particularly important if patients are frail and elderly, because it will help to ascertain whether the family will be able to look after them if required (Cox & Roper, 2005).
- *Occupation*: establish the occupation of patients (or previous occupation if they have been made redundant or have retired). As certain occupations are at risk of particular illnesses, all past occupations should be noted (Gleadle, 2004). For example, construction and associated workers, e.g. electricians, boiler engineers/laggers, may suffer from asbestos-related diseases. Some occupations can be affected by certain diseases, e.g. lorry drivers diagnosed with epilepsy will need to give up their job (Cox & Roper, 2005).
- *Living accommodation*: ascertain where the patient lives and the type of accommodation, e.g. a bungalow, house with an upstairs bathroom, block of flats etc., as this could be pertinent, both as a contributing factor to the presenting complaint and as a consideration when discharging the patient.
- *Travel history*: nowadays, with illnesses such as malaria and severe acute respiratory syndrome (SARS), a travel history is essential (Shah, 2005b), particularly if infection is suspected.
- *Patients' hobbies/interests*: having a knowledge of these allows a clinician to understand patients better and to determine what is important to them (Shah, 2005b).

Smoking and alcohol

It is important to establish patients' current and past smoking and alcohol history because both are implicated in many illnesses:

- *Smoking*: ask patients if they smoke; if they do, confirm details of what they smoke, i.e. cigarettes, cigars or a pipe, including quantity and how long they have been a smoker; if patients do not smoke, but have smoked previously, again confirm details of what they smoked, i.e. cigarettes, cigars or a pipe, the quantity, for how long and when they gave up.
- *Alcohol*: ask patients if they drink alcohol; use the standard unit as a measure (Box 1.3). As there is a tendency to underestimate

Box 1.3 Units of alcohol in common drinks

1 pint of ordinary strength beer – 2 units.
1 pint of ordinary strength cider – 2 units.
1 pub measure of spirit – 1 unit.
1 glass of wine – 2 units.
1 alcopop – 1.5 units

(Source: Department of Heath, 2008)

alcohol intake, separate weekdays and weekend intake should be established, together with any history of binge drinking (remember to include wine taken with meals, as this is often forgotten) (Shah, 2005b). Adopt a non-judgemental approach, but get to the point; for example, 'how much alcohol do you normally drink?'; if there is no clear answer, 'how much did you drink in the last week/fortnight?' (Shah, 2005b).

Patients' ideas, concerns and expectations

An appropriate and sound history taking technique will help to identify patients' ideas, concerns and expectations. Effective communication techniques (listed above) are paramount. The most common cause of patient dissatisfaction following a consultation is a failure in communication (Ford *et al.*, 2005). To avoid this situation, it is helpful to:

- Thank patients for their cooperation.
- Ask patients if there is anything else they would like to say.
- Provide a short summary outlining the patient's problem or symptoms – this will help to confirm a mutual understanding, reducing the risks of a misunderstanding.

(Shah, 2005b)

SYMPTOMS OF DISEASE

A symptom can be defined as an indication of a disease or disorder noticed by the patient (a sign is an indication of a particular disease or disorder that is observed during clinical examination)

(McFerran & Martin, 2003). A comprehensive and effective history taking technique will help elicit the patient's symptoms (see pp. 19–20).

Each symptom must be analysed methodically following the 'TINA' system approach (see pp. 20–21 for a more detailed explanation):

- **T**iming – onset, duration, pattern, progression.
- **I**nfluences – precipitating, aggravating and relieving factors.
- **N**ature – character, site, severity, radiation, volume.
- **A**ssociations – any other associated signs and symptoms.

(Source: Ford *et al.*, 2005)

The main symptoms of disease are:

- Pain.
- Dyspnoea.
- Palpitations.
- Ankle oedema.
- Syncope.
- Dizziness.
- Headache.
- Dysphagia.
- Nausea and vomiting.
- Change in bowel habit.
- Abdominal pain.

These symptoms are discussed at length in Chapter 2.

AN OVERVIEW TO CLINICAL EXAMINATION

Having completed history taking, a differential diagnosis will be possible, which will help to direct the focus of the clinical examination (Ford *et al.*, 2005). A suggested approach to clinical examination is now described.

Preparation

- Obtain the patient's consent (Nursing and Midwifery Council, 2008b).

- Assemble any necessary equipment and aids required for the examination.
- Adhere to local infection control protocols as appropriate, e.g. wear appropriate clothing and wash and dry hands (Box 8.1, see pp. 197–198).
- Ensure privacy: screen the bed or couch.
- Consider the need for a chaperone, who should be of the same gender as the patient (Thomas & Monaghan, 2007). The patient has a right to request a chaperone when undergoing any procedure or examination; where intimate procedures or examinations are required, nurses should ensure that they are aware of any cultural or religious beliefs or restrictions the patient may have, which may prohibit the procedure being performed by a member of the opposite sex (Nursing and Midwifery Council, 2008a).
- Clear the left side of the bed (right side of the patient): always perform examination from the left side of the bed (Cox & Roper, 2005) (unless left-handed, in which case approach from the right), as this will provide a feeling of control over the situation (Thomas & Monaghan, 2007).
- Expose the area that needs to be examined (avoid embarrassing the patient): ensure that there are no draughts and close any open windows if necessary. It is important that the patient does not get cold during the examination: shivering will cause muscle sounds which will interfere with auscultation (Ford *et al.*, 2005).
- Position the patient appropriately on the couch/bed: initially, this will be sitting at an angle of 45° for examination of the cardiovascular system; the position will usually be changed for other aspects of the examination, e.g. for examination of the abdomen, the patient will need to be in a supine position. Sometimes the positioning of the patient will be determined by the patient's condition. For example, if patients are very breathless, they will probably need to sit at 90°; if they are unconscious, they will be supine throughout the examination.

- Ensure that the hands are warm before examining the patient: palpating using cold hands can result in the abdominal muscles contracting, impairing examination (Ford *et al.*, 2005).

Procedure for clinical examination

The procedure for clinical examination can be broken down into bodily systems, the format for this book. These bodily systems should be examined in turn:

- Cardiovascular system (Chapter 3).
- Respiratory system (Chapter 4).
- Gastrointestinal and genitourinary systems (Chapter 5).
- Neurological system (Chapter 6).
- Musculoskeletal system (Chapter 7).

The examination of each system should encompass the following:

- Inspection (looking).
- Palpation (feeling).
- Percussion (tapping).
- Auscultation (listening).

(Box 1.4) (Thomas & Monaghan, 2007)

Box 1.4 Principles of examination

Inspection:

- Look at the whole patient.
- Check there is adequate lighting.
- Look around the bed for clues, e.g. nebulizer, sputum pot.
- Look carefully and thoroughly.
- Look for abnormalities.

Palpation:

- Check whether the patient has any tenderness or pain.
- Initially palpate lightly and gently, then palpate firmly.
- Check for the presence of thrills.

Continued

Percussion:

- Percuss and compare both sides (listen and feel for any differences).

Auscultation:

- Ensure appropriate positioning of the patient to optimize sounds.
- Compare abnormalities with the norm.

(Source: Gleadle, 2004)

Although described separately in different chapters, the examination routines for each system should not be considered as entirely separate entities: when examining several systems at once, a single fluid routine should be used throughout the clinical examination.

Following clinical examination

Following clinical examination, it is important to:

- Thank patients for their help and co-operation.
- Invite and answer any questions they may have.
- Ensure that the examination routine is formally closed, so that the patient knows that it has finished.
- Leave the patient in a comfortable position and not exposed.
- Ensure appropriate documentation is made (Nursing and Midwifery Council, 2008b) (Chapter 9).

TESTS AND INVESTIGATIONS

Try to follow the sequence history taking, clinical examination and then tests and investigations when seeing a patient; a common mistake is to rush into investigations before considering the history or clinical examination (Stride & Scally, 2005).

When ordering tests and investigations, it is easy to mindlessly order a whole range of them. However, there are many problems with this approach:

- Investigations cannot be used in isolation – is the X-ray finding or blood test result relevant or an incidental finding?
- Investigations can be inaccurate – there can be problems with technique, reagents or interpretation of the findings.
- Investigations pose risks – radiation exposure, unnecessary further procedures, and so on.
- Investigations can be costly to the patient and to society.

(Stride & Scally, 2005)

Therefore, after history taking and clinical examination, order or perform tests and investigations relevant to the case (Beasley *et al.*, 2005).

CONCLUSION

This chapter has provided an overview to history taking and clinical examination. The objectives of history taking have been listed and how to establish a rapport with the patient has been described. The sequence of history taking, together with symptoms of disease, has been discussed. An overview to clinical examination has been provided.

REFERENCES

Beasley R, Robinson G, Aldington S (2005) From medical student to junior doctor: the scripted guide to patient clerking. *Student BMJ* **13**: 397–440.

Cox N, Roper T (2005) *Clinical Skills: Oxford Core Text*. Oxford University Press, Oxford.

Department of Health (2008) *Unit Calculator*. Available at www. dh.gov.uk [accessed on 30 June 2008].

Ford M, Hennessey I, Japp A (2005) *Introduction to Clinical Examination*. Elsevier, Oxford.

Gleadle J (2004) *History and Examination at a Glance*. Blackwell Publishing, Oxford.

Marcovitch H (2005) *Black's Medical Dictionary*, 41st edn. A & C Black, London.

McFerran T, Martin E (2003) *Mini-Dictionary for Nurses*, 5th edn. Oxford University Press, Oxford.

Nursing and Midwifery Council (NMC) (2008a) *Chaperoning*. Available at www.nmc-uk.org [accessed on 26 January 2008].

Nursing and Midwifery Council (NMC) (2008b) *The Code: Standards of Conduct, Performance and Ethics for Nurses and Midwives*. NMC, London.

Shah N (2005a) Taking a history: introduction and the presenting complaint. *Student BMJ* **13**: 314–315

Shah N (2005b) Taking a history: conclusion and closure. *Student BMJ* **13**: 358–359

Stride P, Scally P (2005) Better ways of learning. *Student BMJ* **13**: 360–361

Thomas J, Monaghan T (2007) *Oxford Handbook of Clinical Examination and Practical Skills*. Oxford University Press, Oxford.

Symptoms of Disease

2

Gareth Walters

INTRODUCTION

A symptom can be defined as an indication of a disease or disorder noticed by the patient; a sign is an indication of a particular disease or disorder that is observed during clinical examination (McFerran & Martin, 2003).

Eliciting and analysing the patient's symptoms are an integral part of clinical assessment. Symptoms should be compared with signs. For example, on examination, ankle oedema (swelling) may be evident, but during history taking the patient may complain of pain in the lower legs during walking; the former is a sign, the latter is a symptom. Therefore, it is important to recognize the difference between the two, not only to structure clinical assessment, but also to understand when symptoms and signs may be related and part of the same diagnosis.

The aim of this chapter is to provide an understanding of the symptoms of disease.

LEARNING OUTCOMES

At the end of this chapter, the reader will be able to:

❏ Discuss strategies to elicit the patient's symptoms.
❏ Outline the analysis of the patient's symptoms.
❏ Describe common symptoms.

STRATEGIES TO ELICIT THE PATIENT'S SYMPTOMS

When eliciting the patient's symptoms, it is important to follow a structured approach. An open question, such as 'what is the problem that has brought you to hospital?', is a good start which lets the patient describe what they feel is the most important symptom. This can then be followed by a series of closed questions (often requiring yes or no answers) to explore the symptom further. For example, if the patient initially answers 'I have a pain in my chest', questions such as 'how long have you had it?' and 'what makes it worse?' will encourage the patient to elaborate. Negative answers are just as important when filtering out irrelevant information.

It is important to try to avoid 'leading questions', as some patients, in their efforts to try to be helpful, may 'lead you up the garden path'.

ANALYSIS OF THE PATIENT'S SYMPTOMS

The patient's symptoms can be analysed systematically following the 'TINA' approach:

- Timing – onset, duration, pattern, progression.
- Influences – precipitating, aggravating and relieving factors.
- Nature – character, site, severity, radiation, volume.
- Associations – any other associated signs and symptoms.

(Source: Ford *et al.*, 2005)

Timing

It is important to establish when the symptom began, how it began (i.e. sudden or gradual onset), whether it is continuous or intermittent and whether it is improving or getting worse. If it is intermittent, the length of each episode should be established.

Influences

It is important to establish whether any factors influence the symptom. Are there any precipitating factors? Does anything aggravate the symptom? What makes it worse? What relieves it? For example, if the patient has ischaemic heart disease, exercise could induce or worsen chest pain, whereas rest could relieve it.

Nature

It is important to establish the nature of the symptom and whether it is mild or severe. For pain, the site, radiation, character (ache, dull, stabbing, burning, etc.), severity (pain score), mode and rate of onset, duration, frequency, associated symptoms and exacerbating/relieving factors should be determined (Thomas & Monaghan, 2007).

Associations

It is important to establish whether there are any other associated signs and symptoms.

COMMON SYMPTOMS

Pain

Pain is an unpleasant sensory and emotional experience associated with actual or potential tissue damage or described in terms of such damage (Marcovitch, 2005). It is the body's way of alerting the patient that there is something wrong. It can range from mild discomfort to excruciating distress (McFerran & Martin, 2003). If the patient is in pain, it is important to identify the cause, to evaluate its impact on the patient, to plan a treatment strategy and to assess the effects of treatment (Swash & Glynn, 2007).

There are common features to all pain assessment regardless of which of the body's systems is the cause. To illustrate this fact, chest pain is used, but the same approach to pain assessment can be applied to abdominal pain, headache, etc.

Site and character

There are many varieties and causes of chest pain (Table 2.1). Central chest pain, in particular, should always be taken very seriously. Angina pectoris is a pain in a band across the front of the chest, often described as a tightness or an ache. In the case of myocardial infarction, the pain is more severe and can be crushing in nature. Pleuritic chest pain can occur anywhere across

Table 2.1 Common causes of chest pain

Type of chest pain	Cause
Cardiac chest pain	Angina pectoris (ischaemic heart disease)
	Myocardial infarction
	Acute pericarditis
Respiratory chest pain (pleuritic)	Pulmonary embolism
	Pneumothorax
	Pneumonia (pleurisy)
Gastrointestinal pain	Oesophageal spasm
	Oesophageal reflux disease
	Peptic ulcer
	Trapped wind
Musculoskeletal pain	Fractured rib
	Intercostal muscle strain
	Costochondritis
Cardiorespiratory collapse (severe central chest pain)	Massive pulmonary embolism
	Tension pneumothorax
	Acute aortic dissection

the chest, often at the lung bases or across the lateral chest. A comparison between angina pectoris and pleuritic pain is given in Table 2.2.

Gastrointestinal pain is described as retrosternal, i.e. it feels as if it originates from behind the breastbone. It is continuous, often accompanied by epigastric pain. Pain described as 'indigestion' or 'dyspepsia' is a burning sensation, but gastrointestinal pain can also be an ache similar to angina, or severe pain mimicking myocardial infarction. Musculoskeletal pain is localized to a rib or intercostal muscle and tends to be sharp in character and anywhere on the chest. Costochondritic pain is at the site of rib insertions at the sternum. It tends to be 'reproducible' on palpation.

Radiation

Angina and myocardial infarction pain can radiate to the jaw, left arm and shoulder. Pleuritic pain is localized and usually does not radiate. Gastrointestinal pain often radiates through to the back, particularly in the case of a peptic ulcer, and can mimic cardiac pain by radiating to the jaw.

Table 2.2 Comparison of angina pectoris and pleuritic chest pain

Characteristic	Angina pectoris	Pleuritic chest pain
Site	Central chest	Localized, often lateral chest
Onset	On exertion, cold weather or with stress	Acute or sudden
Severity	An ache	Can be severe and sharp
Character	A tightness across chest or a central chest ache	Sharp pain that catches on inspiration
Radiation	To jaw and left shoulder and arm	No radiation
Progression	Constant ache whilst exertion maintained	Worsens or crescendos before help is sought
Relieving factors	Stopping exertion, nitrate (GTN) spray	Shallow breathing
Exacerbating factors	Further exertion	Deep inspiration
Associated symptoms	Breathlessness, palpitations, nausea	Productive cough, breathlessness, haemoptysis

Severity

All chest pain can mimic the pain of myocardial infarction in severity; even trapped wind or musculoskeletal pain can be sufficiently severe to make the patient very distressed and anxious.

A patient having a myocardial infarction often describes the pain as '10 out of 10', or the worst pain ever experienced. Angina pectoris is an ache that becomes more severe on exertion. Other causes of severe central chest pain that must be considered are pulmonary embolism, pneumothorax and aortic dissection.

Onset

Angina can occur during exercise, stress or cold weather, whereas unstable angina or myocardial infarction can cause pain at rest. Pleuritic pain with a sudden onset is suggestive of pulmonary embolism or pneumothorax, whereas pleuritic pain with a gradual onset is suggestive of pneumonia (pleurisy).

Sudden onset of pain following eating or drinking is suggestive of oesophageal spasm or reflux. Musculoskeletal pain is usually only present on movement, but costochondritis (inflammation of rib cartilage) can be present at rest.

Duration and progression

Angina is usually brought on by exercise and is relieved by rest; it persists or worsens if exertion is continued. Pain from myocardial infarction is not relieved by rest and persists until the patient receives effective treatment, e.g. intravenous morphine.

Pleuritic pain often persists beyond successful treatment of a chest infection and either reaches a crescendo or fluctuates in severity from day to day. Musculoskeletal pain is usually severe at first and improves with time; the pain associated with costochondritis increases over time.

Relieving and exacerbating factors

Angina is worse in cold weather and relieved by rest or sublingual glyceryl trinitrate (GTN). The pain of myocardial infarction is constant and not relieved by GTN.

The sharp and constant central chest pain associated with acute pericarditis is relieved by sitting forward and is worsened when lying flat. Pleuritic pain is worse on deep inspiration, and so the patient tends to take shallow breaths to relieve it.

Musculoskeletal pain is worse on movement and palpation. Oesophageal pain is often worse with fatty food and relieved by taking antacids or peppermint water.

Associated features

Angina often appears as an isolated symptom, but can be associated with breathlessness and palpitations on exertion. Myocardial infarction pain is accompanied by sweating, nausea and vomiting and a feeling of impending doom. Pleuritic pain may be accompanied by breathlessness at rest or on exertion, productive or dry cough and haemoptysis.

Gastrointestinal pain can be accompanied by other gut symptoms, such as nausea, vomiting or diarrhoea. Musculoskeletal pain is usually isolated but, in the case of costochondritis, features of inflammation are associated. These features will be picked up when undertaking a review of systems in the history.

Dyspnoea

Dyspnoea can be defined as difficulty in breathing or breathlessness (Marcovitch, 2005). The patient may report feeling 'short of breath' or 'out of puff'. On examination, breathlessness is an objective sign with a high respiratory rate (>20 breaths/min) and possibly low oxygen levels (hypoxia). Some patients who describe themselves as being breathless may not actually be breathless on examination.

Most causes of dyspnoea are cardiac or respiratory related (Table 2.3), but it can be a manifestation of systemic disease or

Table 2.3 Common causes of breathlessness

Type	Cause
Cardiac	*Acute*
	Pulmonary oedema (heart failure)
	Myocardial infarction
	Chronic
	Valve disease, e.g. aortic stenosis
	Chronic heart failure
Respiratory	*Acute*
	Asthma
	Pulmonary embolism
	Pneumonia
	Pneumothorax
	Chronic
	Chronic obstructive pulmonary disease
	Pulmonary fibrosis
	Chest wall disease
Systemic disease	Severe anaemia
	Thyrotoxicosis
	Anxiety
Metabolic acidosis (hyperventilation)	Severe sepsis
	Diabetic ketoacidosis

metabolic acidosis in severe disease. Cardiac causes of breathlessness are characterized by:

- Orthopnoea.
- Paroxysmal nocturnal dyspnoea.

Orthopnoea is breathlessness when the patient is lying flat, i.e. the patient has to sleep propped up in bed or in a chair (McFerran & Martin, 2003). Fluid accumulates in the lungs when in the supine position (pulmonary oedema), and increased dyspnoea, associated with closure of the upper airway, can heighten anxiety about lying flat. Asking the patient how many pillows are needed when asleep provides a good measure of the severity of orthopnoea (normally only one pillow is needed).

Paroxysmal nocturnal dyspnoea can also occur when fluid accumulates in the lungs. As awareness of this decreases when asleep, large amounts of fluid can accumulate in the lungs, resulting in the patient suddenly waking up gasping for breath and frightened; sitting over the edge of the bed or standing up often provides immediate relief. Breathlessness is often accompanied by wheezing, known as 'cardiac asthma'; this is caused by oedema of the airways rather than the bronchospasm of asthma, and can be accompanied by coughing up white or pink, frothy, blood-stained sputum.

Severity of breathlessness

Asking patients about their exercise limitations can help to assess the severity of breathlessness. For example:

- What makes them breathless? Climbing flights of stairs? If so, how many?
- How far can they walk on the flat, and up a hill?
- Do they get breathless getting dressed or bending over?
- Do they have oxygen at home to help them?

The New York Heart Association (NYHA) grades breathlessness according to exercise limitation (Remme & Swedberg, 2001).

Table 2.4 The New York Heart Association (NYHA) grading
of breathlessness (Adapted from Remme & Swedberg, 2001)

NYHA grade	Exercise limitation
1	No breathlessness on exertion
2	Breathless on severe exertion
3	Breathless on mild exertion
4	Breathless at rest

It provides a good measure of functional disability and the ability
to carry out the activities of daily living. Physicians also use this
scale to determine the prognosis in a variety of cardiac conditions.
The grades are shown in Table 2.4.

Palpitations

Palpitations can be defined as a forcible and/or irregular beating
of the heart, such that the patient is conscious of its action (Marcovitch, 2005). Unfortunately, palpitations mean different things to
different people. They may represent an awareness of one's own
heart beating, extra or missed beats, or a sensation of a consis-
tently fast or slow heart rate. For most patients, the more serious
palpitations are caused by bradycardia (heart rate <60 beats/min)
or tachycardia (heart rate >100 beats/min). Missed or extra beats
are called ectopic (extrasystolic) beats.

It is important to ask patients what they mean by palpitations.
Asking patients to tap the rhythm on the table with their fingers
is a useful tool to determine whether the rate is normal, slow, fast
or very fast, and also whether it is regular or irregular. Normal
heart rate and rhythm are called normal sinus rhythm and can be
confirmed on a 12-lead electrocardiogram. Paroxysmal palpitations, usually tachycardias, are short periods of fast palpitations lasting minutes to hours, either regular or irregular, which
begin and end abruptly. Close questioning will elicit these
details, indicating the probable need to investigate with a 24-h
electrocardiogram.

Ankle oedema

Oedema can be defined as an abnormal accumulation of fluid beneath the skin, or in one or more bodily cavities (Marcovitch, 2005). Although fluid can accumulate in any area of soft tissue, most people are mobile and gravity dictates that the fluid collects most noticeably in the ankles. If more severe, this can progress up the thighs and abdomen.

Mobility is reduced and the patient can complain of leg swelling or aching, particularly noticeable at the end of the day. If a patient is more immobile or bed bound, fluid can collect in the lower back (sacrum) and in the groin, which can go unnoticed unless specifically looked for on examination.

Right or congestive cardiac failure is by far the most common cause of ankle oedema; the patient should be asked questions about underlying heart disease and specifically about other symptoms of heart disease. However, diseases with large fluid shifts (cirrhosis, renal nephrotic syndromes) and nutritional lack of protein (hypoalbuminaemia) can also produce significant oedema.

Oedema in a single limb usually represents local disease, e.g. inflammation caused by allergy or infection (cellulitis), or a blockage as in lymphoedema or deep vein thrombosis (DVT).

Syncope

Syncope can be defined as a fainting episode caused by a drop in blood pressure, resulting from either a reduction in cardiac output or decreased peripheral vascular resistance (Marcovitch, 2005). The brain is reliant on cardiac output for perfusion of the brainstem and maintenance of consciousness. Cardiac output is determined by the heart rate and blood pressure. Failure of either of these can cause failure of perfusion and momentary or long-standing loss of consciousness. Common causes of syncope are listed in Table 2.5.

When talking about a syncopal episode, the term 'collapse' is best avoided. Collapse provides very little information about the incident or event and, in itself, is not a diagnostic term; it does

Table 2.5 Common causes of syncope

Type of syncope	Description	Cause
Vaso-vagal syncope (simple faint)	Sudden onset, grey and clammy Lightheadedness and nausea Loss of consciousness with bradycardia and low blood pressure Slow recovery over a few minutes	Unpleasant stimuli: pain, blood or heat
Cardiac syncope (Stokes–Adams attacks)	Sudden blackout with no warning May be preceding palpitations Thready pulse Sudden recovery with flushing	Tachyarrhythmia or bradyarrhythmia: sustained or paroxysmal Obstructive structural heart lesions: cardiomyopathy, valve stenoses
Postural syncope	Lightheadedness and syncope on standing from sitting or lying	Autonomic neuropathy: diabetes mellitus, Parkinson's disease Carotid hypersensitivity Low blood volume
Neurological syncope	Often a preceding aura Associated features of urinary incontinence and tongue biting Blackout or classic fit syndrome	Fit (epilepsy) Drop attacks: brainstem stroke
Other	Syncope on certain events	Cough syncope Micturition syncope

not describe whether patients have had a blackout and fallen to the floor unconscious, or whether they have tripped over or fallen to the floor because of a lower limb musculoskeletal problem.

It is important to distinguish between a seizure (or fit) with loss of consciousness, a sudden blackout without warning and a fall with subsequent head injury and loss of consciousness. The usual problem is that the patient remembers very little about the episode, and so an eye witness account from a family member or from the ambulance crew is of paramount importance.

Tachy- or bradyarrhythmias, such as ventricular tachycardia or slow atrial fibrillation, can lead to reduced blood pressure and brain perfusion. Paroxysmal arrhythmias can cause sudden syncope, termed a Stokes–Adams attack (cardiac syncope). There is no warning (aura), but once adequate circulation returns, the patient becomes flushed and consciousness returns. Ask a bystander about the episode and enquire about paroxysmal palpitations and heart disease. These episodes can also occur in patients with structural heart problems, such as aortic stenosis, where the valve area is narrowed and cardiac output is reduced, particularly on exertion.

Postural hypotension is blood pressure that falls on standing from a lying position, causing sudden lightheadedness and syncope. It usually occurs in elderly patients, particularly those with diabetes mellitus or Parkinson's disease. However, it can be observed in any patient who has moderate blood or fluid loss, e.g. gastrointestinal bleed or severe dehydration. Ask patients if they become lightheaded or black out when standing up. A good reference point is when they get out of bed in the morning or in the night to go to the bathroom.

Neurological syncope is also common. Transient ischaemic attacks are small strokes that last for less than 24 h and can cause episodic blackouts, called sudden drop attacks, if the stroke affects the blood supply to the brainstem. A seizure can cause syncope. There are a variety of epilepsy syndromes, but a generalized tonic–clonic (*grand mal*) seizure is the most common, causing loss of consciousness. The classic presentation is of a vague aura or warning of an impending fit. The whole body becomes rigid or tonic for up to 1 min and the patient falls to the ground, often suffering head or limb injury. The tongue is usually bitten and there is usually incontinence of urine. The clonic phase is a generalized convulsion which involves rhythmic jerking of the muscles lasting for about 1 min. Usually the fit is self-limiting, but can persist for several hours or until help is sought and the patient is treated with sedatives. As the patient will not remember the episode, a collateral account is necessary from a bystander. The patient may remember the preceding aura.

Dizziness

Dizziness is a vague term for a variety of symptoms, and so the presenting complaint requires detailed clarification. Vertigo is a sensation or, an illusion of movement, usually rotational or tipping, where a patient feels that the room is spinning. It is very unpleasant because it is not related to movement, can be present when lying flat and is usually accompanied by nausea and vomiting. Causes of vertigo include diseases of the ear (e.g. Ménière's disease), the vestibular system (acute labyrinthitis) or neurological diseases of the brainstem and VIIIth cranial nerve (vestibulocochlear). Careful history and eliciting other ear, nose and throat neurological symptoms, such as headache, tinnitus and deafness, can point towards a specific cause.

Lightheadedness still sounds vague, but ascertaining whether the patient means this will exclude vertigo as a symptom. The best way to describe this is altered consciousness with a feeling of almost passing out, often associated with a visual disturbance. This is why this type of dizziness is called pre-syncope. It follows that the common significant causes of lightheadedness are cardiac and neurological, exactly the same as for syncope!

Lightheadedness on exertion could have a cardiac cause, because cardiac output is put under pressure during exercise and any deficiencies will be exaggerated, or a respiratory cause, because the patient becomes short of oxygen (hypoxic) and starts to hyperventilate and blow off carbon dioxide. This can cause pre-syncope.

Panic and anxiety have a variety of effects on the conscious state from hyperventilation lightheadedness to an altered sense of reality (de-realness and de-personalization), where the patient feels disconnected from the surrounding world, lost in an anxious state.

Headache

Headache is a very common symptom in healthcare practice and varies in its presentation and in its potential to represent serious underlying disease. History is of paramount importance in order to recognize serious intracranial pathologies. The majority of headaches represent benign problems. Headaches can be acute or chronic and, like any pain, the site, character and nature should be established immediately as they can point to the pathology. The common causes of acute and chronic headaches are shown in Table 2.6, and Table 2.7 provides the characteristics of acute headache.

Most headaches lasting for more than a few hours are attributed to muscle tension, and can persist or recur over days and weeks. Most often described is a band-like ache or a pressure around the whole anterior part of the head. Recurrent acute pains that are localized to the forehead or below the eyes, with localized tenderness on deep palpation, can be ascribed to sinusitis, particularly with other symptoms of upper respiratory tract disease.

It is a myth that high blood pressure in itself causes headaches, but malignant hypertension, an acute acceleration of blood pres-

Table 2.6 Common causes of acute and chronic headaches

Type of headache	Cause
Acute headache	Subarachnoid haemorrhage
	Acute sinusitis
	Tension headache
	Migraine
	Malignant hypertension
	Meningitis and encephalitis
	Sudden increase in intracranial pressure caused by intracranial haemorrhage
	Temporal arteritis
	Cluster headache
Chronic headache	Tension headache
	Raised intracranial pressure
	Chronic sinusitis
	New refractive prescription (spectacles)

Table 2.7 Characteristics of acute headache

Diagnosis	Characteristic of headache
Subarachnoid haemorrhage	Sudden onset, severe and persistent occipital 'thunderclap' headache. Often described as the worst headache ever experienced. Usually followed by vomiting, drowsiness and focal neurological signs
Acute meningitis	A non-specific headache, but increasingly severe and persistent and part of a clinical triad of fever, neck stiffness and headache that develops over a few hours
Temporal arteritis (giant cell arteritis)	Severe unilateral temporal headache with scalp or temporal tenderness. Usually accompanied by pain in jaw on chewing
Tension headache	A tight band sensation, throbbing or 'bursting' sensation or pressure behind the eyes. Particularly at times of stress. Can also have pain and tenderness in the muscles at the back of the neck. Not associated with any neurological signs
Cluster headache	Recurrent episodes of acute excruciating unilateral pain that clusters around one eye. Men more than women in their 20 s and 30 s. Can be provoked by alcohol
Classical migraine	Throbbing unilateral headache preceded by an aura of visual disturbance lasting for 15–60 min; nausea and vomiting can occur

sure with damage to the retina and optic nerve and kidneys, can cause an acute headache. The most serious chronic headache to recognize is that of rising intracranial pressure. Any growing lesion occupying space in the skull, such as a tumour or an abscess, causes an increase in intracranial pressure and a characteristic headache that is worse in the morning after waking and worse on coughing, straining or bending over. It is accompanied by vomiting and blurred or reduced vision, and should be taken seriously with consideration of urgent computed tomography imaging of the brain.

Dysphagia

Dysphagia is difficulty in swallowing (Marcovitch, 2005). It is an important symptom to recognize because it often represents serious underlying pathology. First, it is necessary to distinguish what the patient means by difficulty in swallowing. Does it occur at the mouth or throat? Or is it a sensation of something sticking further down behind the sternum?

Ask about dysphagia to solids and liquids. Oesophageal motility disorder (achalasia) causes a long history of dysphagia to both solids and liquids with regurgitation. Food sticking at the back of the throat or choking may be caused by poor swallowing mechanisms following a stroke affecting the bulbar nerves, and therefore the coordination and movement of muscles in the mouth and throat (bulbar palsy), or by a pharyngeal pouch. Acute pharyngitis and tonsillitis cause pain and difficulty in swallowing as a result of inflammation.

Progressive dysphagia to solids and then, eventually, liquids suggests an enlarging growth caused by oesophageal or gastric cancer. This can be a result of a benign stricture, but the patient requires urgent investigation, particularly if there is significant weight loss and other alimentary symptoms. Ask about weight loss and appetite.

Nausea and vomiting

Nausea is a feeling of wanting to vomit, often accompanied by sweating, pallor and abdominal discomfort. Vomiting is the expulsion of gastric contents via the mouth. These are very non-specific symptoms.

Common causes are not necessarily related to local gastric disease (Table 2.8). A good general history should elicit the probable origin. Consider acute infections, particularly urinary tract infections and flu-like illnesses, metabolic disease (diabetic keto-acidosis, uraemia) and central nervous system disease. There is a vomiting centre in the medulla oblongata of the brain, called the chemoreceptor trigger zone (CTZ); consider diseases such as meningitis, migraine and raised intracranial pressure. Nausea and vomiting are common side-effects of drug therapy, particularly opiates, e.g. morphine and codeine, and chemotherapeutic and immunotherapeutic agents (British Medical Association and Royal Pharmaceutical Society of Great Britain, 2007).

Table 2.8 Common causes of nausea and vomiting

Type	Cause
Gastrointestinal	Acute gastroenteritis
	Acute gastritis
	Appendicitis
	Reflux oesophagitis
	Bowel obstruction
	Constipation
	Acute pancreatitis
Drug side-effects	Opiates
	Chemotherapeutic agents
Metabolic	Urinary tract infection
	Acute renal failure
	Addison's disease
	Diabetic ketoacidosis
Neurological	Cerebellar disease
	Migraine
	Raised intracranial pressure
	Subarachnoid haemorrhage
	Head injury
Miscellaneous	Pregnancy
	Myocardial infarction
	Inner ear disease: vertigo, Ménière's disease
	Acute glaucoma
Psychiatric	Bulimia nervosa
	Alcohol abuse

Many gastrointestinal diseases can cause nausea and vomiting, and are often accompanied by other alimentary symptoms, such as dyspepsia, dysphagia, bloating, diarrhoea, constipation and abdominal pain.

Ask specifically about the presence of blood in vomit. Vomiting fresh blood (haematemesis) signifies an upper gastrointestinal bleed (above the level of the duodenum). It is important to quantify how long this has been going on and the amount of blood present in each vomit. Any more than 300 ml of fresh blood is considered to be a large bleed and the patient may need resuscitation and urgent endoscopy. Also ask about the presence of blood in the gastrointestinal tract in other guises. Coffee-ground vomit is altered blood that has sat in the stomach for a few hours, but

Table 2.9 Causes and sites of upper gastrointestinal haemorrhage

Site	Cause
Oesophagus	Liver cirrhosis related to oesophageal varices
	Mallory–Weiss tear secondary to vomiting
	Oesophageal cancer
	Reflux oesophagitis
Stomach and duodenum	Peptic ulcer
	Gastric cancer
	Acute gastritis
	Erosions

also signifies an upper gastrointestinal bleed. As does melaena, which is tarry stools containing altered blood that has passed through the alimentary tract. Common causes of upper gastrointestinal haemorrhage are listed in Table 2.9.

Change in bowel habit

Normal bowel habits vary from person to person. Some people have naturally quicker transit times than others, and therefore there is a large variation in what is normal. A patient's perception of constipation and diarrhoea varies: constipation may mean infrequent passage of stools (less than twice a week), passage of hard stools or straining or incomplete evacuation, whereas diarrhoea may mean watery or loose stools, the presence of blood in stools, a large frequency of stools passed in rapid succession, urgency to defaecate or passage of a stool accompanied by bloating or abdominal discomfort. About 25% of the population have an altered bowel habit at some time, but only a small percentage have serious underlying pathology. Common causes of constipation and diarrhoea are listed in Table 2.10 and Box 2.1, respectively.

Abdominal pain

Abdominal pain, often ill-defined and sometimes very unpleasant for the patient, has a variety of different causes (Table 2.11). The characteristics of pain have already been discussed, and time

Table 2.10 Common causes of constipation

Type	Cause
Colon or rectum	Colon obstruction by cancer, volvulus or stricture
	Slow colonic motility, particularly in patients with a history of chronic laxative abuse
	Hirschsprung's disease
Dietary insufficiency	Inadequate water intake
	Inadequate fibre intake
	Overuse of coffee, tea and alcohol
Systemic disease	Hypothyroidism
	Diabetic autonomic neuropathy
	Spinal cord injury
	Head injury
	Stroke
	Multiple sclerosis
	Parkinson's disease
Drugs	Opiates
	Iron supplements
	Calcium-channel blockers
	Anticholinergic agents

Box 2.1 Common causes of diarrhoea

- Overflow diarrhoea in constipation.
- Inflammatory bowel disease: Crohn's disease and ulcerative colitis.
- Infective enteritis: *Clostridium difficile* infection, viral gastroenteritis, bacterial gastroenteritis, food poisoning.
- Irritable bowel syndrome.
- Small bowel malabsorption: coeliac disease, tropical sprue, chronic pancreatitis.
- Food allergy: lactose intolerance.
- Anxiety and stress.
- Post-gastrectomy.
- Hyperthyroidism.
- Chemotherapeutic drugs.

---

spent eliciting these features cannot be overstated. When assessing abdominal pain, the two most helpful features are character and site. The abdomen can be divided into segments (see p. 102).

Table 2.11 Causes of acute abdominal pain by anatomical region

Region	Cause
Epigastrium	Acute or chronic pancreatitis
	Peptic ulcer
	Reflux oesophagitis
Left upper quadrant	Hypersplenism
	Splenic rupture
Right upper quadrant	Acute or chronic hepatitis
	Biliary colic
	Acute cholecystitis
Loins	Renal colic
	Acute pyelonephritis
Left and right lower quadrants	Acute diverticulitis (left)
	Constipation
	Ruptured ovarian cyst
	Ectopic pregnancy
	Caecal cancer (right)
	Acute appendicitis (right)
	Mesenteric adenitis (right)

Pain from the major abdominal organs corresponds to their anatomical position. Abdominal maps can be used to describe the location of pain. For example, liver pain with hepatitis is felt in the right upper quadrant. Pain from splenic rupture is felt in the left upper quadrant, and bladder pain is felt in the suprapubic area.

Pain from parts of the gastrointestinal tract or 'gut' is produced by a different mechanism, and is a direct result of the embryological origin of the nerve supply to the gut. Simplistically, the area of the abdominal wall in which the pain is felt corresponds to the area of gut which has the same embryological origin as that area of the abdomen. As there are no pain receptors in the gut itself, the pain is referred to these other areas.

The foregut is the first and upper part of the gut, from the mouth to the mid-part of the duodenum where the bile duct joins the gut. The midgut represents the bowel from the mid-duodenum to the transverse colon, two-thirds of the way across. The hindgut continues from the transverse colon to the anus. With that in mind, pain from the stomach, e.g. a peptic ulcer, is felt (or 'referred') across the upper abdomen, pain from the appendix at the colonic caecum is felt across the mid-abdomen or umbilical area, and pain from the sigmoid colon is felt across the lower abdomen.

Gut pain is called 'colic'. Colic is a deep cramping ache that comes and goes in increasing intensity with gut peristalsis. It is poorly localized, as already described, and the patient finds it difficult to get comfortable. At this stage, there is little clue as to the cause of the pain without further history and a period of observation.

Peritonitis is a more specific pain felt at the site of the problem. It is caused by inflammation or irritation of the peritoneum at a particular site. Unlike the bowel itself, the peritoneum has pain receptors, and so any pain felt is immediately localized. The character is different: it is severe, continuous and tends to be a sharper pain than colic. It rises steadily in intensity until help is sought. If the patient stays very still, some relief can be obtained.

Peritonitis occurs when part of the gut is inflamed or obstructed (as in acute appendicitis or cholecystitis) and presses on the peritoneum. In the case of peritonitis from appendicitis, pain is felt in the right lower quadrant. Therefore, the classic picture of appendicitis is of a few hours or days of mid-abdominal colic, followed by a localization of the pain to the right lower quadrant as the appendix becomes more inflamed and the peritoneum becomes irritated.

Complete perforation of a hollow organ in the abdomen, such as a perforated gastric ulcer or sigmoid colon, causes generalized peritonitis, and the pain is severe and widespread. Biliary colic is pain from the bile duct that causes crescendos of severe pain in the right upper abdomen, and sometimes through to the upper back and right shoulder. The pain relates to the obstruction of the passage of bile and can be associated with eating fatty foods. Other symptoms are nausea, vomiting and diarrhoea.

Renal colic is slightly exceptional as the kidneys are retroperitoneal organs, i.e. behind the posterior peritoneum that separates them from the other abdominal organs. Renal colic is caused by blockage of the ureters, usually by renal stones. Ureteric peristalsis produces a characteristic colic pain in the loins that radiates around the flanks to the lower abdomen and into the groin. It is usually unilateral and the patient is unable to get comfortable.

CONCLUSION

Eliciting and analysing a patient's symptoms are integral to clinical assessment. In this chapter, strategies to elicit the patient's symptoms and their analysis have been discussed. Common symptoms have been listed and described in detail.

REFERENCES

British Medical Association and Royal Pharmaceutical Society of Great Britain (2007) *British National Formulary*, 53rd edn. BMJ Publishing, London.

Ford M, Hennessey I, Japp A (2005) *Introduction to Clinical Examination*. Elsevier, Oxford.

Marcovitch H (2005) *Black's Medical Dictionary*, 41st edn. A & C Black, London.

McFerran T, Martin E (2003) *Mini-Dictionary for Nurses*, 5th edn. Oxford University Press, Oxford.

Remme W, Swedberg, K (2001) Guidelines for the diagnosis and treatment of chronic heart failure. *Eur Heart J* **22**: 1527–1560.

Swash M, Glynn M (eds) (2007) *Hutchison's Clinical Methods*, 22nd edn. W. B. Saunders, Edinburgh.

Thomas J, Monaghan T (2007) *Oxford Handbook of Clinical Examination and Practical Skills*. Oxford University Press, Oxford.

Examination of the Cardiovascular System

3

INTRODUCTION

The cardiovascular system is the term used to describe the whole circulatory system: the heart, the systemic circulation (arteries, veins and capillaries) and the pulmonary circulation (Marcovitch, 2005). It can be compromised by several common and potentially life-threatening diseases, in particular coronary artery disease and congestive cardiac failure (Cox & Roper, 2005).

The aim of this chapter is to provide an understanding of the examination of the cardiovascular system.

LEARNING OUTCOMES

At the end of this chapter, the reader will be able to:

❑ List the symptoms associated with diseases of the cardiovascular system.
❑ Discuss the peripheral examination of the cardiovascular system.
❑ Describe the procedure for non-invasive blood pressure measurement.
❑ Discuss the measurement of jugular venous pressure.
❑ Outline inspection and palpation of the precordium.
❑ Outline auscultation of the heart.
❑ Discuss the examination of the vascular system in the lower limbs.

SYMPTOMS ASSOCIATED WITH DISEASES OF THE CARDIOVASCULAR SYSTEM

Symptoms associated with diseases of the cardiovascular system include:

- Chest pain.
- Breathlessness.
- Orthopnoea.
- Paroxysmal nocturnal dyspnoea.
- Ankle swelling.
- Palpitations.
- Collapse.
- Exercise intolerance.

PERIPHERAL EXAMINATION OF THE CARDIOVASCULAR SYSTEM

To undertake an examination of the cardiovascular system, the patient should ideally be on a couch (or similar) lying at an angle of 45° and exposed from the waist up.

Inspection

- Note the immediate environment of the patient: e.g. presence of glyceryl trinitrate (GTN) spray on the bedside locker, cardiac monitor, infusion pumps and oxygen masks (Ford *et al.*, 2005).
- Observe the patient's general appearance: note the presence of breathlessness, distress or anxiety.
- Examine the patient's hands: assess temperature and colour; observe for signs of poor peripheral perfusion, e.g. pale or cyanosed peripheries, cool in temperature; check the capillary refill time (Figure 3.1).
- Observe for finger clubbing (Figure 4.1, see p. 80): thickening and broadening of the fingertips that can be associated with certain chronic respiratory and cardiac diseases (Marcovitch, 2005).
- Observe for splinter haemorrhages (bleeding under the fingernails that could indicate endocarditis) (Marcovitch, 2005),

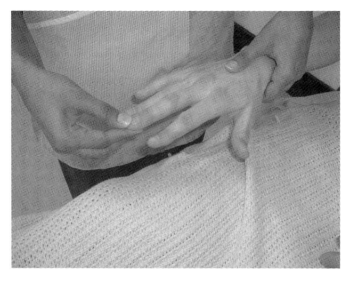

Fig 3.1 Checking the capillary refill time

yellowish tar staining (indicating a smoker) and tendon xan-thomata (indicating raised cholesterol) (Ford *et al.*, 2005).

- Observe for cyanosis of the tongue (central cyanosis).
- Observe for malar flush (reddening of the cheeks with a bluish tinge caused by dilation of the capillaries in the cheeks secondary to pulmonary hypertension): can be associated with mitral stenosis.
- Observe around the patient's eyes for the presence of xantha-lesmata: small yellowish papules (small solid elevations of the skin) suggestive of high cholesterol.
- Observe for corneal arcus: a grey ring around the iris suggestive of high cholesterol.
- Check for anaemia: using the index finger, gently pull down the right lower eyelid to expose the conjunctiva; the anterior aspect of the conjunctiva is normally a brighter red colour than the posterior aspect; in anaemia, there is no distinction (Cox & Roper, 2005).

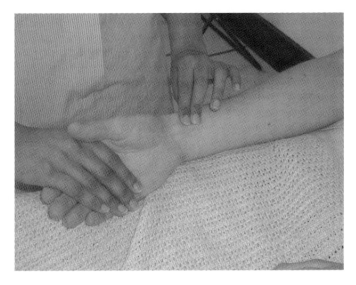

Fig 3.2 Checking the radial pulse

Assessment of pulses

- Assess the patient's radial pulses.
- Hold the patient's right hand and palpate the radial pulse using the tips of the index and middle fingers (the pulse can be felt on the radial aspect of the flexor surface of the forearm, a few centimetres proximal to the wrist) (Figure 3.2) (Cox & Roper, 2005).
- Count the rate of the pulse: e.g. using a watch with a second hand, count the number of beats in 30 s and multiply this by two; care should be taken if the pulse is irregular; a normal pulse rate is considered to be between 60 and 100 beats/min, a tachycardia is a pulse rate of >100 beats/min and a brady-cardia is a pulse rate of <60 beats/min (Resuscitation Council UK, 2006).
- Assess the rhythm of the pulse: is it regular or irregular (the rate usually quickens during inspiration – sinus arrhythmia)?;

an irregular pulse is usually caused either by ectopic beats or atrial fibrillation.

- Palpate both radial pulses together and compare: differences between the two may indicate acute aortic dissection or proximal arterial disease (Cox & Roper, 2005).
- Compare the apex beat with the radial pulse and check for a pulse deficit (in atrial fibrillation, the heart rate is sometimes faster than the pulse, the difference being termed the 'pulse deficit').
- Assess the volume of the pulse: a rapid, weak, thready pulse is a characteristic sign of shock; a full bounding or throbbing pulse may be indicative of anaemia, heart block, heart failure or the early stages of septic shock.
- Check for a collapsing pulse (sign of aortic regurgitation): using the palm of the left hand, grasp the patient's right distal forearm and elevate (Figure 3.3); a vibrating pulse felt in the fingers indicates a collapsing pulse.

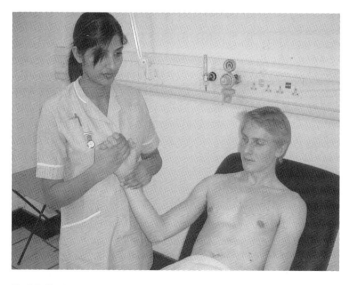

Fig 3.3 Checking for a collapsing pulse

- Compare central (femoral or carotid) and distal (radial) pulses: a discrepancy in the volume between them could be caused by a fall in cardiac output (and also cold ambient temperature).
- Compare radial and femoral pulses: a delay in the femoral pulse may indicate coarctation of the aorta.

Assessment of perfusion
Capillary refill time

Decreased skin perfusion is often characterized by cool peripheries, skin mottling, pallor, cyanosis and delayed capillary refill (>2 s). The following procedure is suggested for the assessment of capillary refill (Figure 3.1):

- Explain the procedure to the patient.
- Elevate the extremity, e.g. digit, slightly higher than the level of the heart (this will ensure the assessment of arteriolar capillary and not venous stasis refill).
- Blanch the digit for 5 s and then release; a sluggish (delayed) capillary refill (>2 s) may be caused by circulatory shock, pyrexia or a cold ambient temperature.

NON-INVASIVE BLOOD PRESSURE MEASUREMENT

Of all the measurements routinely undertaken in clinical practice, the recording of the blood pressure is potentially the most unreliably and incorrectly performed (British Hypertension Society, 2006a). It is essential that blood pressure recordings are accurate and reliable: good practice can significantly reduce measurement errors and help to ensure that the blood pressure recording is accurate and reliable.

Approximately 40% of adults in England and Wales have hypertension (this percentage increases with age), a significant risk factor for stroke, chronic renal failure and coronary heart disease [National Institute for Clinical Excellence (NICE) & British Hypertension Society, 2006].

Systolic and diastolic blood pressure

Systolic blood pressure: peak blood pressure in the artery following ventricular systole (contraction).

Diastolic blood pressure: level to which the arterial blood pressure falls during ventricular diastole (relaxation).

(Talley & O'Connor, 2001)

Korotkoff's sounds

Five different sound phases, known as 'Korotkoff's sounds' (Korotkoff, a Russian surgeon, first described the auscultation method of measuring blood pressure in 1905), can be heard as the blood pressure cuff is slowly released:

- Phase 1: a thud.
- Phase 2: a blowing or swishing noise.
- Phase 3: a softer thud than in phase 1.
- Phase 4: a disappearing blowing noise.
- Phase 5: silence.

(Sources: Talley & O'Connor, 2001;
Dougherty & Lister, 2004)

Practically, the systolic reading is when Korotkoff's sounds are first heard and the diastolic reading is when the sounds disappear (British Hypertension Society, 2006a).

Which arm?

The blood pressure should initially be measured in both arms, and the arm with the higher readings should be used for subsequent measurements [Beevers *et al.*, 2001; Medicines and Healthcare Products Regulatory Agency (MHRA), 2006; NICE & British Hypertension Society, 2006]. Although a difference in blood pressure measurements between the arms can be expected in 20% of patients, if this difference is more than 20 mmHg for systolic or more than 10 mmHg for diastolic on three consecutive readings, further investigation is probably indicated (MHRA, 2006; NICE & British Hypertension Society, 2006).

Procedure for manual measurement of blood pressure

The traditional manual blood pressure device (Figure 3.4) using auscultation is still a very popular and, when used correctly, reli-

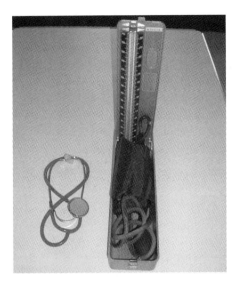

Fig 3.4 Traditional manual blood pressure device

able method of recording blood pressure. The following procedure for its use is recommended:

- Ideally, ensure that the patient has been sitting or lying down for at least 5 min and is comfortably relaxed.
- Check the equipment, ensuring that it is in good working order.
- Explain the procedure to the patient and obtain consent.
- Ask the patient to remove any tight clothing from around the arm.
- Ensure that the patient's arm is supported at the level of the heart. If the arm is unsupported, the blood pressure is likely to be erroneously increased as a result of muscle contraction in the arm (Smith, 2003). If the arm is higher than the level of the heart, this can lead to an underestimation of the diastolic pressure by as much as 10 mmHg (MHRA, 2006).

- Select an appropriately sized cuff: the bladder of the cuff should encircle at least 80% of the arm, but no more than 100%.
- Place the cuff snugly onto the patient's arm, with the centre of the bladder over the brachial artery: most cuffs have a 'brachial artery indicator', an arrow which can be aligned with the brachial artery.
- Position the manometer close to the patient: it should be vertical and at the nurse's eye level.
- Ask the patient to refrain from talking or eating during the procedure as this can result in an inaccurate higher blood pressure (McAlister & Straus, 2001).
- Estimate the systolic pressure: palpate the brachial artery, inflate the cuff and note the reading when the brachial pulse disappears; then deflate the cuff.
- Inflate the cuff to 30 mmHg above the estimated systolic level which was required to occlude the brachial pulse. Approximately 5% of the population have an auscultatory gap; this is when Korotkoff's sounds disappear just below the systolic pressure and reappear above the diastolic pressure (Figure 3.5) (Talley & O'Connor, 2001). Estimating the systolic pressure will help to ensure that the cuff is sufficiently inflated to record an accurate systolic pressure.
- Palpate the brachial artery.
- Place the diaphragm of the stethoscope gently over the brachial artery. Avoid applying excessive pressure on the diaphragm and do not tuck the diaphragm under the edge of the cuff, because either of these actions could partially occlude the brachial artery, delaying the occurrence of Korotkoff's sounds (Dougherty & Lister, 2004).
- Open the valve and slowly deflate the cuff at a rate of 2– 3 mmHg/s, recording when Korotkoff's sounds first appear (systolic) and disappear (diastolic).
- Document the systolic and diastolic blood pressure readings on the patient's observation chart following local protocols.

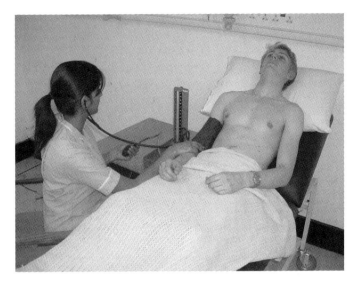

Fig 3.5 Checking the patient's blood pressure

Compare with previous readings and inform the nurse in charge/medical team as appropriate.

(Source: British Hypertension Society 2006a, b;
NICE & British Hypertension Society, 2006)

Errors in blood pressure measurement

Errors in blood pressure measurement can occur for several reasons, including:

- Defective equipment, e.g. leaking tubing or a faulty valve.
- Failure to ensure that the mercury column reads 0 mmHg at rest.
- Too rapid deflation of the cuff.
- The use of an incorrectly sized cuff: if it is too small, the blood pressure will be overestimated and, if it is too large, the blood pressure will be underestimated.
- Cuff not at the same level as the heart.

- Failure to observe the mercury level properly: the top of the mercury column should be at eye level.
- Poor technique (e.g. failing to note when the sounds disappear).
- Digit preference: rounding the reading up to the nearest 5 or 10 mmHg.
- Observer bias, e.g. expecting a young patient's blood pressure to be normal.

(Source: British Hypertension Society, 2006a)

Automated blood pressure devices

When automated blood pressure devices (Figure 3.6) were first manufactured, their accuracy and reliability were questioned (Beevers *et al.*, 2001). However, improved technology has led to the development of more accurate and reliable devices (Beevers *et al.*, 2001), some of which have been tested and approved for use by the British Hypertension Society (2006a).

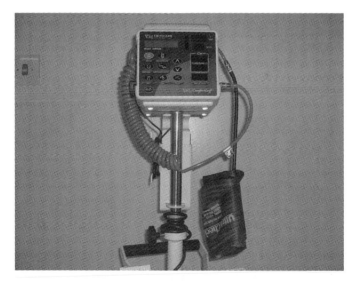

Fig 3.6 Automated blood pressure device

Most automated devices measure blood pressure using one of the following techniques:

- Oscillometry to detect arterial blood flow (most commonly used device).
- A microphone to detect Korotkoff's sounds.
- Ultrasound to detect arterial blood flow.

(British Hypertension Society, 2006a)

Procedure for automated measurement of blood pressure

The principles for the accurate measurement of blood pressure using an automated electronic device are similar to those for the manual recording of blood pressure using a sphygmomanometer with regard to patient preparation, patient position and cuff choice/placement (Dougherty & Lister, 2004). However, when using an automated electronic device, it is important to be familiar with its workings and to follow the manufacturer's recommendations.

MEASUREMENT OF JUGULAR VENOUS PRESSURE

The jugular venous pressure can be defined as the blood pressure in the jugular veins (Cook, 1996; McFerran & Martin, 2003). The internal jugular vein is observed to assess the central venous pressure which correlates with the right atrial pressure (Scott & MacInnes, 2006). The most common cause of a raised jugular venous pressure is congestive cardiac failure: the raised venous pressure reflects right ventricular failure (Epstein *et al.*, 2003).

Pressure in the right atrium is an important indicator of cardiac or pulmonary disease; as the right atrium communicates directly with the right internal jugular vein, the pressure within the vein provides an accurate indication of right atrial pressure (Cox & Roper, 2005). When the pressure in the right atrium is sufficiently high, blood flows back into the internal jugular vein. This can be observed as a pulsation, which enables the clinician to estimate the pressure in the atrium (Talley & O'Connor, 2001).

Related anatomy and physiology

The jugular veins, which drain blood from the head, have two sets of branches, internal and external:

Internal jugular vein: lies deep in the root of the neck (Cox & Roper, 2005), medial to the sternomastoid muscle (Figure 3.7). It communicates directly with the superior vena cava and the right atrium, without any intervening valves (Epstein *et al.*, 2003), i.e. there are no valves between the right atrium of the heart and the internal jugular vein.

External jugular vein: lies lateral to the sternomastoid muscle and is more superficial than the internal jugular vein; it is therefore easier to see (Cox & Roper, 2005).

Although the external jugular vein can be identified more easily than the internal jugular vein, it can become compressed as it enters the chest, and therefore cannot be relied upon to assess the position or waveform of the jugular venous pressure (Talley & O'Connor, 2001).

Normal jugular venous pressure

The mean pressure in the right atrium is normally less than 7 mmHg (9 cmH$_2$O); as the sternal angle is situated approximately 5 cm above the right atrium, the normal jugular pressure pulse should not be more than 4 cm (9 cm minus 5 cm) above the sternal angle (Figure 3.8) (Douglas *et al.*, 2005). Therefore, in a healthy patient with normal right atrial pressure:

- *Sitting at a 45° angle*: the transition point between the distended vein and the collapsed vein may or may not be visible; if it is visible, the pulsation will be seen just above the clavicle.
- *Lying flat*: the jugular vein will be distended and the pulsation will not be visible.
- *Sitting upright*: the upper part of the vein will be collapsed and the transition point between it and the distended vein will be obscured, i.e. the pulsation will not be seen.

(See Figure 3.8) (Douglas *et al.*, 2005)

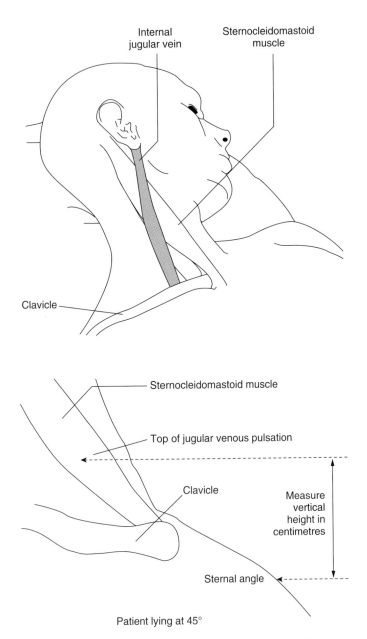

Fig 3.7 Anatomy of the jugular veins and measuring the height of jugular venous pressure

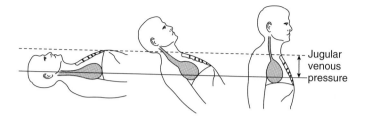

Fig 3.8 Effect of patient position on jugular venous pressure

Jugular venous pressure waveform

Practitioners experienced in assessing the jugular venous pressure can gain further detailed information by scrutinizing the jugular venous pressure waveform (Scott & MacInnes, 2006). The jugular venous pressure waveform varies during the cardiac cycle; there are three stages in which the pressure increases (known as the A, C and V waves) and two stages in which it decreases (known as X and Y descent). Cox & Roper (2005) is a useful resource for further information.

'Cannon waves'

In atrioventricular dissociation (atrial and ventricular contractions are not related in time), the right atrium sometimes contracts against a closed tricuspid valve, resulting in large jugular venous pulsations or 'cannon waves'; these 'cannon waves' occur at irregular intervals because sometimes the tricuspid valve will be shut and sometimes it will be open (Cox & Roper, 2005). Atrioventricular dissociation can be seen in third degree (complete) atrioventricular block and ventricular tachycardia.

Distinguishing between jugular venous pulsation and the carotid pulse

The jugular venous pulsation can be distinguished from the carotid pulse because it is:

- Visible, but not palpable.
- Moves with respiration (decreases on inspiration).
- Affected when pressure is applied to the abdomen.

(Ford *et al.*, 2005)

Causes of a raised jugular venous pressure

The causes of a raised jugular venous pressure include:

- Congestive heart failure.
- Right-sided heart failure.
- Cardiac tamponade.
- Pulmonary embolism.
- Obstruction of superior vena cava, e.g. tumour.
- Intravenous fluid overload.

(Epstein *et al.*, 2003)

Procedure

- Explain the procedure to the patient.
- Ensure that there is adequate lighting.
- Adopt a position on the patient's right side.
- Whilst ensuring privacy and maintaining the patient's dignity, expose the upper chest. Remove any restrictive clothing from around the patient's neck and chest (McConnell, 1998).
- Position the patient at an angle of 45° to the horizontal, leaving one pillow under the head.
- Ask the patient to turn the head to the left (Figure 3.9).
- Observe the level of the jugular venous pulsations just above the clavicle (Scott & MacInnes, 2006).
- Measure the vertical distance (cm) between the sternal angle (manubriosternal joint or angle of Louis) and the highest visible level of jugular vein pulsation (Figure 3.10) (McConnell, 1998). The normal measurement is less than 4 cm (Scott & MacInnes, 2006); add 5 cm to the measurement because the right atrium is 5 cm below the sternal angle, i.e. the normal measurement is less than 9 cm in total, which equates to the normal pressure in the right atrium (see above).

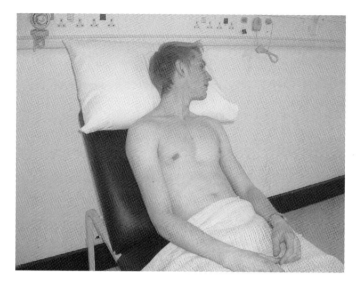

Fig 3.9 Measuring the jugular venous pressure 1: position the patient at an angle of 45° to the horizontal, leaving one pillow under the head, and ask the patient to turn the head to the left

- If there is difficulty seeing the jugular venous pulsation, shine a bright light directly onto the patient's neck (McConnell, 1998).
- If there is still difficulty in seeing the jugular venous pulsation, or if there is uncertainty whether the pulsation seen is venous or arterial, some authorities recommend gentle compression on the right upper quadrant of the abdomen (Figure 3.11): this will transiently increase the venous pressure, resulting in a more prominent internal jugular vein. Venous pulsation usually returns to normal after a few seconds (even with continued abdominal pressure), but, if it remains elevated, this suggests right-sided heart failure (Cox & Roper, 2005). Arterial pulsations are not affected by abdominal compression. For further information, see Cox & Roper (2005).
- Document the findings, i.e. whether the jugular venous pulsation is visible and, if it is, whether it is normal or elevated.

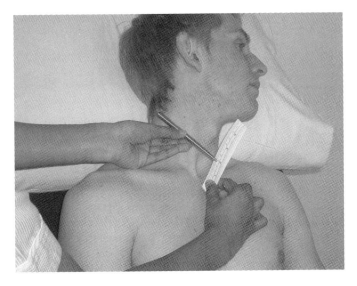

Fig 3.10 Measuring the jugular venous pressure 2: measure the vertical distance (cm) between the sternal angle (manubriosternal joint or angle of Louis) and the highest visible level of jugular vein pulsation

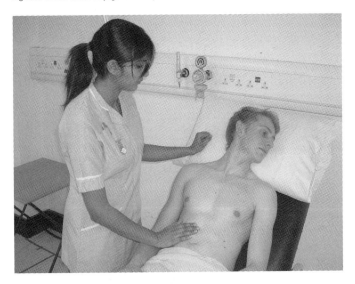

Fig 3.11 Measuring the jugular venous pressure 3: if there is still difficulty in seeing the jugular venous pulsation, or if there is uncertainty whether the pulsation seen is venous or arterial, gentle compression on the right upper quadrant of the abdomen may be helpful

INSPECTION AND PALPATION OF THE PRECORDIUM

The precordium

The precordium is the front of the chest wall over the heart (Cox & Roper, 2005). Of particular importance when inspecting and palpating the precordium is the apex/mitral area (left fifth inter-costal space, mid-clavicular line), as this is where the apex beat can usually be felt (and where mitral valve sounds are best auscultated) (Cox & Roper, 2005).

Cardiac surgery-related scars on the precordium

When inspecting the precordium, it is important to look for scars suggesting previous cardiac surgery. A mid-line sternotomy suggests, for example, a coronary artery bypass graft or valve replacement (Longmore *et al.*, 2007); a left submammary thoracotomy scar suggests mitral valvotomy (Douglas *et al.*, 2005). It is also important to note whether the patient has an implantable pacemaker or cardiovertor/defibrillator; a scar will be visible just below the left (occasionally right) clavicle and, in a thin person, a bulge in the skin may be visible.

Chest deformity

It is important to note any signs of chest deformity, as this can affect the subsequent examination of the heart. For example, pectus carinatum ('pigeon chest') or pectus excavatum ('funnel chest') can displace the heart, thus affecting palpation and auscultation of the precordium (Douglas *et al.*, 2005).

Apex beat

The apex is the tip or summit of an organ (McFerran & Martin, 2003). The apex beat is the impact of the heart against the chest wall during systole (McFerran & Martin, 2003); it is primarily a result of recoil of the apex of the heart as the blood is expelled during systole (Talley & O'Connor, 2001). As it correlates with left ventricular contraction, assessment of the apex beat provides an indication of the functioning of the left ventricle (Scott & MacInnes, 2006).

Sometimes the apex beat is not palpable; this is usually because of a thick chest wall, emphysema, pericardial effusion, shock or dextrocardia (Talley & O'Connor, 2001); rolling the patient into the left lateral position may enable the apex beat to be palpated (Scott & MacInnes, 2006). The location and character of the apex beat should be noted.

Location of the apex beat and causes of displacement

The normal location of the apex beat is the fifth/sixth intercostal space, mid-clavicular line, with the patient lying in a supine position at approximately 45° (Epstein *et al.*, 2003; Scott & MacInnes, 2006). The causes of a displaced apex beat include:

- *Cardiomegaly*: a common cause of the apex beat being displaced inferiorly or laterally.
- *Mediastinal shift*: a large pleural effusion or tension pneumothorax can push the apex beat (and sometimes the trachea) away from the affected side; a collapsed lung can draw the apex beat towards the affected side.
- *Dextrocardia*.

(Sources: O'Neill *et al.*, 1989; Douglas *et al.*, 2005)

Character of the apex beat

Practitioners experienced in cardiac assessment can assess the character of the apex beat. A normal apex beat is short and sharp (Epstein *et al.*, 2003). Abnormal findings of the apex beat include:

Heaving: a sustained and forceful heave caused by an obstruction, e.g. aortic stenosis or systemic hypertension, to the flow of blood out of the heart.

Thrusting: caused by volume overload.

Tapping: felt in mitral stenosis.

Diffuse: left ventricular failure and cardiomyopathy.

(Source: Longmore *et al.*, 2007)

Thrills

Thrills: transmitted heart murmurs – similar to stroking a purring cat (Epstein *et al.*, 2003).

Procedure for inspection and palpation of the precordium

- Explain the procedure to the patient.
- Ensure that the patient is in a supine position at an angle of 45°.
- Whilst ensuring privacy and maintaining the patient's dignity, expose the chest.
- Ask the patient to breathe in and out normally.
- Inspect the precordium for cardiac surgery-related scars (see above). In a female patient, it may be necessary to lift up the left breast to allow full inspection of the precordium. Note any chest shape deformity and unusual pulsations (Scott & MacInnes, 2006).
- Palpate the apex beat (this is usually the fifth/sixth intercostal space, mid-clavicular line) (Figure 3.12) (Scott & MacInnes, 2006): place the right hand, with the fingers outstretched, against the left side of the patient's chest wall and locate the apex beat.
- If locating the apex beat is difficult, roll the patient into the left lateral position. Although this usually makes it easier to locate the apex beat, the lateral position will push the apex beat further outwards because the heart has some degree of mobility in the chest (Epstein *et al.*, 2003).
- Using the tip of a finger, assess the character of the apex beat (see above).
- If the apex beat is displaced, check that the trachea is central (Figure 4.3, see p. 83); if the trachea is deviated, this indicates mediastinal shift (Ford *et al.*, 2005).
- Palpate to the left of the sternum to ascertain whether the hand is lifted with each ventricular contraction (Scott & MacInnes, 2006): place the heel of the right hand with the fingers pointing upwards over the precordium to the left of the sternum (Figure 3.13); in normal circumstances, the movement related to

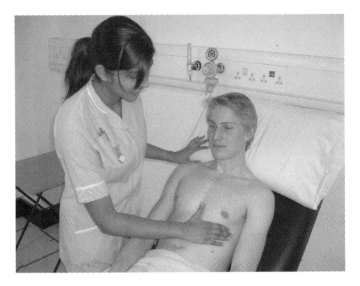

Fig 3.12 Palpate the apex beat (this is usually the fifth/sixth intercostal space mid-clavicular line)

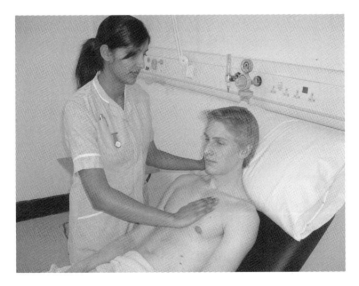

Fig 3.13 Checking for a parasternal heave: place the heel of the right hand with the fingers pointing upwards over the precordium to the left of the sternum

respirations will be felt; if the hand is lifted off the chest with each ventricular contraction, this is referred to as a left parasternal heave, usually caused by right ventricular hypertrophy or volume overload.

AUSCULTATION OF THE HEART

Auscultation can be defined as the action of listening to sounds from the heart, lungs and other internal organs using a stethoscope (Soanes & Stevenson, 2004). Auscultation of the heart is undertaken to establish whether the heart sounds are normal and if there are any additional sounds (Scott & MacInnes, 2006). It is a skill that requires detailed knowledge, practice and experience to ensure competency at distinguishing what is normal and what is abnormal. The priority is to master the recognition of normal heart sounds; it will then be possible to unravel abnormal heart sounds (Cox & Roper, 2005).

There is no consensus as to what constitutes the correct routine for auscultation of the heart (Cox & Roper, 2005); therefore, the key principles of the procedure are described here.

Heart valves

There are four valves in the heart:

- *Mitral valve*: consisting of two triangular cusps, it prevents backflow of blood into the left atrium when the left ventricle contracts.
- *Tricuspid valve*: consisting of three triangular cusps, it prevents backflow of blood into the right atrium when the right ventricle contracts.
- *Aortic valve:* it prevents regurgitation of blood back into the left ventricle following ventricular contraction.
- *Pulmonary valve:* it prevents regurgitation of blood back into the right ventricle following ventricular contraction.

(Marcovitch, 2005)

Normal heart sounds and related physiology

The heart sounds are usually described as 'lub-dup'. The first heart sound ('lub'), which is often referred to as 'S1', is caused by closure of the mitral and tricuspid valves and is best heard at the apex. It corresponds to the beginning of ventricular systole (Waugh & Grant, 2006). Sometimes, splitting of the first heart sound occurs, which is normal.

The second heart sound ('dup'), which is often referred to as 'S2', is slightly higher pitched. It is caused by closure of the aortic and pulmonary valves and is best heard in the second/third intercostal space, at the left sternal edge. It corresponds to the end of ventricular systole and the beginning of atrial systole. Splitting of the second heart sound can occur with inspiration.

After the second heart sound, there is a short gap before the heart sounds of the next cardiac cycle; this is ventricular diastole and signifies the time during which the ventricles are filling with blood (Scott & MacInnes, 2006).

Using a stethoscope

The stethoscope is an instrument used for listening to the sounds produced by the action of the lungs, heart and other internal organs (Marcovitch, 2005). It was introduced into medicine 200 years ago; originally, it was a wooden cylinder with a hole drilled from one end to the other (Epstein *et al.*, 2003). The modern stethoscope has two earpieces, which are connected by tubing to a chest device usually consisting of a bell and a diaphragm. The ear pieces should be angled forwards, i.e. in the same direction as the practitioner's external auditory meatus (Epstein *et al.*, 2003).

The functions of the stethoscope are to:

- Transmit sounds from the patient's chest.
- Exclude extraneous noise.
- Selectively emphasize sounds of certain frequencies, allowing the practitioner to concentrate on them.

(Epstein *et al.*, 2003)

The stethoscope should be used correctly, as the diaphragm and bell each amplify different sounds (Scott & MacInnes, 2006):

- *Diaphragm*: used to detect high-pitched sounds, e.g. S1, S2 and some murmurs; it should be pressed firmly against the skin.
- *Bell*: used to detect low-pitched sounds, e.g. mitral stenosis murmur, and should be placed very lightly against the precordium, otherwise it will effectively be a diaphragm.

(Sources: Cox & Roper, 2005; Scott & MacInnes, 2006)

Standard sites for auscultation

Standard sites for auscultation of the heart are (Figure 3.14):

- *Mitral area*: left fifth intercostal space, mid-clavicular line: this is where the mitral valve sounds are best auscultated.
- *Tricuspid area*: left fourth intercostal space, just lateral to the sternum: this is where the tricuspid valve sounds are best auscultated.
- *Pulmonary area*: left second intercostal space, just lateral to the sternum: this is where the pulmonary valve sounds are best auscultated.
- *Aortic area*: right second intercostal space, just lateral to the sternum: this is where the aortic valve sounds are best auscultated.

(Cox & Roper, 2005; Scott & MacInnes, 2006)

Abnormal heart sounds

During auscultation of the heart, it is important to detect added sounds and murmurs (Longmore *et al.*, 2007), including:

Third heart sound (S3): a low-pitched sound heard just after the second heart sound (S2); the most important pathological cause is left ventricular failure, although it can be a normal finding in healthy young persons and in pregnancy (Cox & Roper, 2005).

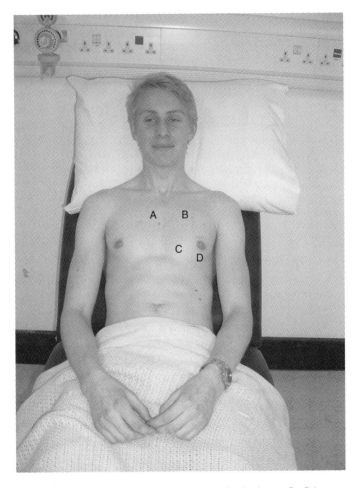

Fig 3.14 Standard sites for auscultation of the heart. A = Aortic area; B = Pulmonary area; C = Tricuspid area; D = Mitral area

Fourth heart sound (S4): a low-pitched sound heard just before the first heart sound (S1); never normal, it indicates a non-compliant ventricle (Cox & Roper, 2005).

Cardiac murmur: characterized by a whooshing or blowing noise. Causes include turbulent blood flow across an abnormal valve, septal defect and outflow obstruction; sometimes it is a normal finding (Douglas *et al.*, 2005). If the murmur is present between the two heart sounds (i.e. between S1 and S2), it is termed a systolic murmur, and, if it is present between each set of two heart sounds (i.e. between S2 and S1), it is termed a diastolic murmur (Scott & MacInnes, 2006). Systolic murmurs are more common and easier to hear than diastolic murmurs (Cox & Roper, 2005).

There are two types of diastolic murmur:

- *Early diastolic murmur*: a high-pitched sound, beginning loudly and then rapidly becoming quieter; most commonly caused by aortic regurgitation. At the beginning of diastole, the pressure in the aorta is at its maximum and then decreases; hence, in aortic valve disease, regurgitation of blood back across the aortic valve can occur particularly at the beginning of diastole when the pressure in the aorta is high.
- *Mid-diastolic murmur*: a low-pitched sound, most commonly caused by mitral stenosis: turbulent flow of blood from the left atrium into the left ventricle across the diseased mitral valve.

(Source: Cox & Roper, 2005)

There are three types of systolic murmur:

- *Pansystolic murmur*: usually a gentle blowing sound heard during systole; most common cause is mitral valve disease: incomplete closure of the mitral valve leads to regurgitation of blood back across the valve during ventricular contraction.
- *Ejection systolic murmur*: usually a harsh sound, the most common cause is aortic stenosis: during left ventricular contraction, blood flow across the diseased aortic valve is turbulent.

- *Late systolic murmur*: usually seen late in systole; often caused by mitral valve prolapse which, if severe, can cause some regurgitation.

(Source: Cox & Roper, 2005)

Pericardial friction rub: has been described as a creaking sound similar to walking on firm snow; caused by pericarditis, it is best heard when patients hold their breath (Ford *et al.*, 2005).

Procedure

Recommendations for auscultation of the heart vary. The following procedure is based on Cox & Roper (2005):

- Explain the procedure to the patient.
- Whilst ensuring privacy and maintaining the patient's dignity, expose the chest.
- Position the patient supine at an angle of 45°.
- Ensure the room is quiet.
- Ask the patient to breathe in and out normally.
- Using the diaphragm, auscultate over the mitral area (Figure 3.14).
- Identify the first (S1) and second (S2) heart sounds; to assist identification of these heart sounds, it may be necessary to palpate the carotid pulse at the same time, as this will coincide with the first heart sound (Ford *et al.*, 2005) (Figure 3.15).
- Ask the patient to roll slightly into a left lateral position and, using the bell, auscultate over the mitral area: this is the best position and method to auscultate the low-pitched mid-diastolic murmur of mitral stenosis.
- Auscultate over the tricuspid area (Figure 3.14) using the bell: this is the optimum position to detect the mid-diastolic murmur of tricuspid stenosis.
- Auscultate over the tricuspid area (Figure 3.14) using the diaphragm: this is the optimum position to detect the pansystolic (i.e. heard throughout systole) murmur associated with tricuspid regurgitation and a pericardial friction rub.

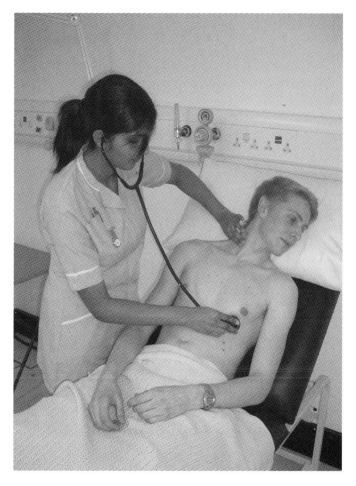

Fig 3.15 Identifying the first (S1) and second (S2) heart sounds; it may be necessary to palpate the carotid pulse at the same time, as this will coincide with the first heart sound

- Auscultate over the pulmonary area (Figure 3.14) using the diaphragm: this is the optimum position to detect pulmonary murmurs; the bell is rarely used at this site.
- Auscultate over the aortic area (Figure 3.14) using the diaphragm: this is the optimum position to detect murmurs associated with aortic stenosis; the bell is rarely used at this site.
- During the time interval between the first and second heart sounds, listen for added heart sounds and murmurs.
- Whilst asking the patient to hold his/her breath, auscultate over each carotid artery: this is to detect carotid bruits and aortic systolic murmurs radiating to the carotid arteries (Figure 3.16) (Ford *et al.*, 2005).
- Ask the patient to sit forward and to hold his/her breath in expiration, and auscultate with the diaphragm of the stethoscope along the left sternal edge: this is to detect a diastolic murmur associated with aortic incompetence (Figure 3.17) (Ford *et al.*, 2005).
- Document the clinical findings in the patient's notes.

(Sources: Cox & Roper, 2005; Ford *et al.*, 2005)

EXAMINATION OF THE VASCULAR SYSTEM IN THE LOWER LIMBS

Examination of the venous system in the lower limbs should always be undertaken. In particular, check for the possible presence of a deep vein thrombosis, including unilateral leg swelling, pain, oedema, tenderness and redness, although sometimes the patient may be asymptomatic (Gleadle, 2004).

- Expose the patient's legs.
- Look at both legs: compare colour, temperature and size.
- Palpate pulses in both limbs: femoral, popliteal, posterior tibial and dorsalis pedis; signs of an ischaemic limb are detailed in Box 3.1.
- Observe for any ankle oedema: note if it is 'pitting', i.e. an impression can be made with a finger, and observe how high it extends up the limb (Thomas & Monaghan, 2007).

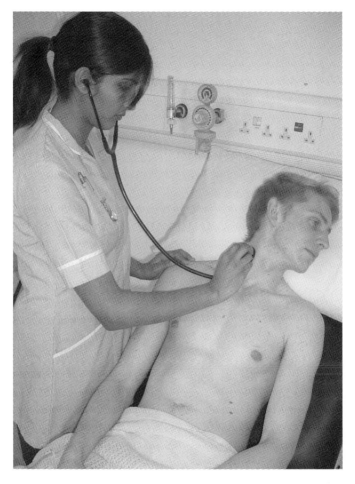

Fig 3.16 Checking for carotid bruits and aortic systolic murmurs radiating to the carotid arteries

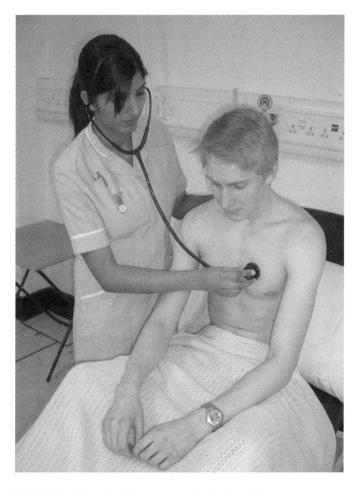

Fig 3.17 Detecting a diastolic murmur associated with aortic incompetence

---

Box 3.1 Signs of acute ischaemia of the lower limb

- Painful (initially).
- Painless (numb).
- Pale.
- Paralysed.
- Pulseless.

(Source: Thomas & Monaghan, 2007)

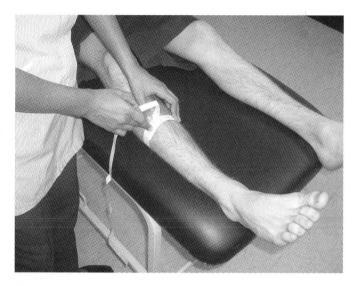

Fig 3.18 Measuring the calf muscle

- Observe for venous distension: check to see whether the superficial veins empty promptly after the limb is elevated (Ford *et al.*, 2005).
- Gently palpate each calf: look for tenderness and warmth; compare both limbs.
- Compare the size of each calf: if one appears to be larger than the other, use a tape measure and compare the circumference

of each calf at a fixed distance from the medial malleolus (Figure 3.18) (Ford *et al.*, 2005).

CONCLUSION

In this chapter, the examination of the cardiovascular system has been described. The examination of the peripheral cardiovascular system and procedures for non-invasive blood pressure measurement have been discussed. The measurement of the jugular venous pressure and auscultation of the heart have been described. Examination of the venous system in the lower limbs has been discussed.

REFERENCES

Beevers G, Lip G, O'Brien E (2001) *ABC of Hypertension*, 4th edn. BMJ Books, London.

British Hypertension Society (2006a) *Let's Do It Well*. Available at www.bhsoc.org/pdfs/hit.pdf [accessed on 10 January 2008].

British Hypertension Society (2006b) *Blood Pressure Measurement with Mercury Blood Pressure Monitors*. Available at www.bhsoc.org [accessed on 10 January 2008].

Cook D (1996) Does this patient have abnormal central venous pressure? *J Am Med Assoc* **275**: 8.

Cox N, Roper T (2005) *Clinical Skills: Oxford Core Text*. Oxford University Press, Oxford.

Dougherty L, Lister S (2004) *The Royal Marsden Hospital Manual of Clinical Nursing Procedures*, 6th edn. Blackwell Publishing, Oxford.

Douglas F, Nicol F, Robertson C (2005) *MacLeod's Clinical Examination*, 11th edn. Elsevier, Edinburgh.

Epstein O, Perkin G, Cookson J, de Bono D (2003) *Clinical Examination*, 3rd edn. Mosby, London.

Ford M, Hennessey I, Japp A (2005) *Introduction to Clinical Examination*. Elsevier, Oxford.

Gleadle J (2004) *History and Examination at a Glance*. Blackwell Publishing, Oxford.

Jevon P (2007) Measuring capillary refill time. *Nursing Times* **103**(12): 26–27.

Longmore M, Wilkinson I, Turmezei T, Cheung C (2007) *Oxford Handbook of Clinical Medicine*. Oxford University Press, Oxford.

Marcovitch H (2005) *Black's Medical Dictionary*, 41st edn. A & C Black, London.

McAlister F, Straus S (2001) Evidence based treatment for hypertension – measurement of blood pressure: an evidence based review. *Br Med J* **322**: 908–911.

McConnell E (1998) Assessing jugular venous pressure. *Nursing* **28**(2): 28.

McFerran T, Martin E (2003) *Mini-Dictionary for Nurses*, 5th edn. Oxford University Press, Oxford.

Medicines and Healthcare Products Regulatory Agency (MHRA) (2006) *Medical Device Alert: Blood Pressure Monitors and Sphygmomanometers*. MHRA, London.

National Institute for Clinical Excellence (NICE) & British Hypertension Society (2006) *NICE/BHS Hypertension Guideline Review*. Available at www.bhsoc.org/NICE_BHS_Guidelines. stm [accessed on 28 June 2006].

O'Neill T, Barry M, Smith M, Graham I (1989) Diagnostic value of the apex beat. *Lancet* **1**: 410–411.

Resuscitation Council UK (2006) *Advanced Life Support*, 5th edn. Resuscitation Council UK, London.

Scott C, MacInnes J (2006) Cardiac patient assessment: putting the patient first *Br J Nursing* **15**(9): 502–508.

Smith G (2003) *ALERT Acute Life-Threatening Events Recognition and Treatment*, 2nd edn. University of Portsmouth, Portsmouth.

Soanes C, Stevenson A (2004) *Concise Oxford English Dictionary*, 11th edn. Oxford University Press, Oxford.

Talley N, O'Connor S (2001) *Clinical Examination: a Systematic Guide to Physical Diagnosis*. Blackwell Science, Oxford.

Thomas J, Monaghan T (2007) *Oxford Handbook of Clinical Examination and Practical Skills*. Oxford University Press, Oxford.

Examination of the Respiratory System

4

Gareth Walters

INTRODUCTION

In the UK, chest disease is a common cause of morbidity and mortality. Acute breathlessness is one of the most common causes of admission to hospital, and lung cancer remains the number one killer of all cancers (Cox & Roper, 2005). Examination of the respiratory system requires a methodical approach to ensure that important signs and symptoms are not missed.

The aim of this chapter is to provide an understanding of the examination of the respiratory system.

LEARNING OUTCOMES

At the end of this chapter, the reader will be able to:

❏ List the symptoms of respiratory disease.
❏ Describe the peripheral examination of the respiratory system.
❏ Describe the examination of the chest.

SYMPTOMS OF RESPIRATORY DISEASE

The symptoms of respiratory disease include:

- Cough.
- Breathlessness.
- Haemoptysis.
- Wheeze.
- Pleuritic pain.
- Sputum.

(Sources: Gleadle, 2004; Ford *et al.*, 2005)

PERIPHERAL EXAMINATION OF
THE RESPIRATORY SYSTEM

- Ask the patient if there is any pain or tenderness anywhere on the body before undertaking the examination.
- Expose the patient to the waist in a sitting position on a couch at an angle of 45°; this is easy with an adjustable examination couch. The use of a few pillows may be necessary.

Environment

- Look around the bed for any clues suggesting a respiratory problem, e.g. nebulizer, oxygen inhaler or sputum pot.
- If there is a sputum pot, ascertain that it belongs to the patient (check the name), and look inside and check the consistency and colour of the sputum; yellow or green (purulent) sputum usually indicates a respiratory tract infection; hard 'plugs' of sputum are usually associated with asthma; haemoptysis can be caused by a number of diseases, including carcinoma of the lung and pulmonary embolism (Thomas & Monaghan, 2007).

Characteristic features associated with respiratory disease

- Look for characteristic features associated with respiratory disease that provide a 'spot' diagnosis or clue to an underlying respiratory problem:
  ○ Evidence of cachexia (severe weight loss) associated with lung cancer or severe chronic obstructive pulmonary disease (COPD).
  ○ Obesity, suffused (swollen and bulging) conjunctivae and overt cyanosis (so-called 'blue bloater' syndrome; also called Pickwickian syndrome) seen in COPD and type 2 respiratory failure due to sleep apnoea syndrome.
  ○ Prolonged expiration phase, breathing through pursed lips, splinting and use of accessory muscles including abdominal and intercostal muscles (so-called 'pink puffer' syndrome); these are signs of hyperinflated lungs seen with emphysema.

Respiratory rate

- Calculate the patient's respiratory rate: count the number of breaths in 30 s and double this for the minute rate. The normal respiratory rate is 12–16 breaths/min. Abnormal respiratory rates include:
  - Respiratory rate of more than 18 breaths/min: called tachy-pnoea, and may indicate underlying hypoxia caused by a variety of respiratory problems, e.g. pneumothorax and pulmonary embolism.
  - Respiratory rate of more than 30 breaths/min: indicates severe respiratory distress, and the patient requires urgent assessment. Patients with acute severe asthma, exacerbations of COPD and severe pneumonia often present in respiratory distress, and can decompensate quickly.
  - Respiratory rate of less than 10 breaths/min: represents hypoventilation (inadequate ventilation); causes include sedative drugs, such as opiates and benzodiazepines, leading to depression of ventilation. Beware of the patient presenting with respiratory distress whose respiratory rate falls; this is usually observed when the patient has become fatigued, and can precipitate respiratory arrest; it is often an indication for intubation and mechanical ventilation (Cox and Roper, 2005; Douglas *et al.*, 2005).

For patients not *in extremis*, observe what makes them breathless throughout the examination. Specifically look at factors such as removing the shirt or repeatedly saying '99'. This is a good guide to the level of respiratory function.

Hands

- Inspect the patient's hands and look closely for the following:
  - Finger clubbing (Figure 4.1): seen in a variety of respiratory diseases (see Box 4.1).
  - Tar staining from cigarette smoking: usually seen on the middle and index fingers.

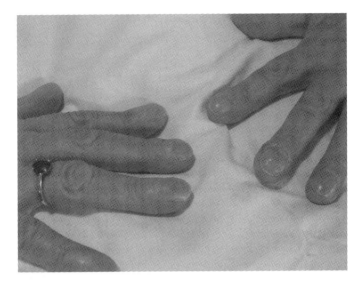

Fig 4.1 Finger clubbing

Box 4.1 Clinical features and respiratory causes of finger clubbing

The clinical features of clubbing are gradual in onset and usually painless:

- Boggy nail bed (the nail moves more freely than a normal nail).
- Increased longitudinal curvature of the nail.
- Loss of the nailfold angle.
- Bulbous fusiform enlargement of the distal digit ('drumsticking').

The respiratory causes of clubbing include:

- Suppurative lung disease: abscess; bronchiectasis; empyema; cystic fibrosis.
- Lung cancer: bronchial carcinoma (non-small cell); mesothelioma.
- Lung fibrosis.

(Adapted from Douglas *et al.*, 2005)

- Peripheral cyanosis: the dusky blue discoloration and mottling of the extremities when hypoxic (caused by the presence of desaturated haemoglobin). It can also occur in cold weather when the circulation is poor, and its presence should precipitate a search for central cyanosis, which does not occur in cold weather and indicates central hypoxia.
- Flapping tremor of carbon dioxide retention.
- β-Agonist (e.g. salbutamol) therapy can cause a fine tremor.

Carbon dioxide retention

Patients with COPD usually retain carbon dioxide (Ward *et al.*, 2006). A flapping tremor is a sign of carbon dioxide retention and may indicate that the patient is acutely ill. It usually consists of course, jerky movements of the wrist.

- Check for the presence of a flapping tremor: ask the patient to outstretch the arms in front, with the wrists cocked and fingers slightly parted (Figure 4.2). Observe for 15 s to establish its absence.

Head and neck

- Ask the patient to open the mouth and put the tongue out and then to the roof of the mouth.
- Look for dusky blue discoloration of the tongue and buccal mucosa, representing central cyanosis. This indicates central oxygen desaturation and blood hypoxia with an increase in deoxygenated haemoglobin (Cox & Roper, 2005).
- Ask the patient to sit forward in order to palpate for cervical lymphadenopathy. Feel the deep cervical and supraclavicular lymph nodes bilaterally. These are most often involved in respiratory disease.
- Look for a raised jugular venous pressure and palpate the ankles for oedema. Many respiratory disorders lead to chronic hypoxia and, in turn, to pulmonary hypertension and right heart failure (Ward *et al.*, 2006). The most common underlying

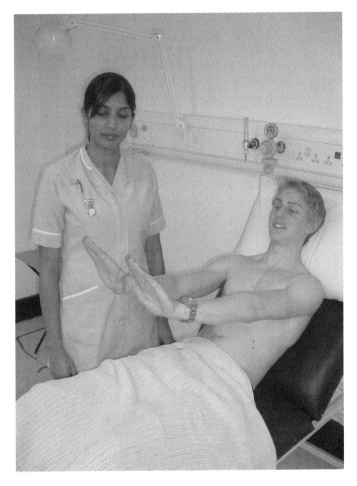

Fig 4.2 Checking for flapping tremor

problem is COPD. Right heart failure manifests as fluid retention and raised jugular venous pressure.

- Palpate the trachea (advise the patient that it will be uncomfortable): place the index finger in the suprasternal notch in the median longitudinal plane and use the middle finger to locate

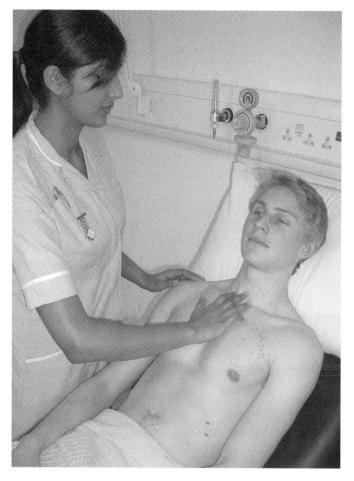

Fig 4.3 Palpation of the trachea

the middle of the tracheal ring (in the longitudinal plane); then slide the index and ring fingers either side of the trachea and decide whether it is central (normal) or deviated to one side (Cox & Roper, 2005) (Figure 4.3). Common causes of tracheal deviation are listed in Box 4.2.

Box 4.2 Common causes of tracheal deviation

Trachea deviating away from the pathology:

- Large pleural effusion.
- Tension pneumothorax.

Trachea deviating towards the pathology:

- Lung fibrosis.
- Lung collapse and consolidation.

- Measure the distance between the sternal notch and the cricoid cartilage: three to four finger breadths in expiration is normal; this is chronically reduced in patients with emphysematous and hyperexpanded lungs.
- Note the presence of a tracheal tug in hyperexpanded lungs: the trachea appears to descend towards the chest cavity on inspiration.

EXAMINATION OF THE CHEST

Inspection of the chest

- Inspect the chest for obvious deformities and characteristic movements of the chest wall at rest:
  - *Thoracic kyphosis*: stooping and increased anterior–posterior curvature of the spine as a result of osteoporotic vertebral destruction; this can lead to breathlessness on exertion and restriction of chest movement. Long-term steroid use, including the use of inhalers, can be the cause.
  - *Scoliosis*: increased lateral curvature of the spine; can result from lung infections and surgery in childhood, and can accompany kyphosis as a manifestation of osteoporosis.
  - *Barrel-shaped chest*: caused by hyperinflation associated with COPD; there is very limited lateral expansion of the lower part of the chest and the thoracic cage moves up on inspira-

tion rather than up and out. This finding is accompanied by the other features of hyperexpansion already discussed.

○ *Asymmetrical chest expansion*: asymmetry between left and right side chest movement; indicates a localized problem in one half of the thorax; this should be confirmed on palpation.

- Inspect for characteristic thoracic scars associated with the presence of chest drains and surgical procedures:

○ *Chest drain insertion scar*: chest drains are inserted for the drainage of pleural effusions and for the aspiration of pneumothoraces generally (Cox & Roper, 2005). Their presence indicates pathology on the same side. If a chest drain is still *in situ*, note whether the drainage bottle contains large amounts of fluid (indicating an effusion) or whether the underwater seal has air bubbling through it (indicating a pneumothorax). After removal, a small 1–2 cm scar will be evident laterally or posteriorly on the affected side of the chest.

○ *Pneumonectomy and lobectomy scars*: pneumonectomy (removal of one lung) and lobectomy (removal of one lobe of the lung) scars are characteristic; indications include removal of a carcinoma and treatment of bronchiectasis where other forms of treatment have failed. Before the use of antibiotics, tuberculosis was sometimes treated surgically by lobectomy or pneumonectomy.

Chest palpation

- Palpate the apex of the heart: the normal position is the fifth intercostal space, mid-clavicular line on the left side. The apex can be difficult to feel or impalpable in COPD, or where there is a large effusion or a pneumothorax. The apex can be deviated (where there may also be tracheal deviation) in an effusion, pneumothorax or lung collapse.

- Assess the symmetry of chest expansion: place the palms of the hands over the upper part of the anterior chest walls (Figure 4.4). The chest should rise equally with each inspiration.

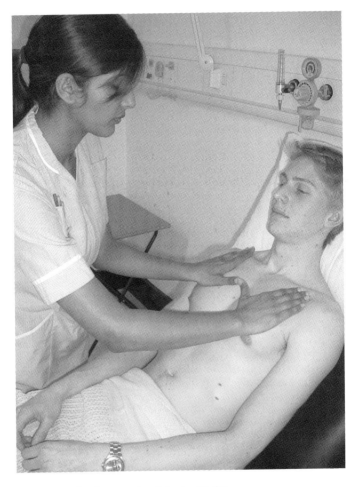

Fig 4.4 Assessing the symmetry of chest expansion

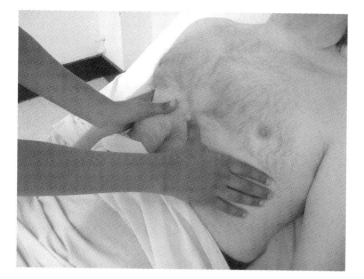

Fig 4.5 Assessing the degree of chest expansion

- Assess the degree of chest expansion: grip the chest symmetrically with the fingertips in the lower rib spaces on either side so that the thumbs touch in the middle in a horizontal straight line (Douglas *et al.*, 2005) (Figure 4.5). Assess chest expansion at the lung bases on either side. Approximate (in centimetres) or note that lateral chest expansion is reduced on a particular side. A tape measure can be used to assess the distance of finger spread if precise measurements are required. Assessment of the degree of chest expansion may confirm earlier findings of chest asymmetry.

Chest percussion

Percussion is the technique of examination of part of the body by tapping it with a finger or an instrument and evaluating the resultant vibrations (McFerran & Martin, 2003). Chest percussion creates a sound (resonance) and palpable vibration that are useful in evaluating underlying lung tissue and the size of internal organs. It is an integral part of any complete examination of the respiratory system; it can provide invaluable information relating to the status of the lungs and can be helpful in determining the position of organs and the presence of masses or fluid (Ford *et al.*, 2005). Chest percussion has few clinical implications unless it is considered with other clinical findings, when it can help with the diagnosis.

Percussion can also be used to evaluate the movement of the diaphragm during respiration. The level of dullness will descend downwards during inspiration (the right side is normally slightly higher than the left) (Epstein *et al.*, 2003).

Percussion should be gentle: do not percuss more heavily than is necessary, as it can be uncomfortable for the patient and will not provide any additional information (Epstein *et al.*, 2003). Achieving a loud tone does not ensure quality; it is more important to obtain different tones and recognize their significance. The force of the tap should be from the wrist, not the forearm or shoulder. The tip of the phalanx should be used, not the finger pads, as this could alter the percussion notes generated (short fingernails are paramount).

The chest can be divided into three zones on each side: upper, middle and lower (Figure 4.6). This provides specific areas for percussion (and auscultation), and also allows abnormal findings to be simply and efficiently described in relation to anatomy.

- Explain the procedure to the patient. This is particularly important because, if the patient is anxious, the chest wall muscles may become tense, which may alter the percussion sound generated.
- Ensure a quiet environment. Noise will make an accurate interpretation of the findings more difficult.

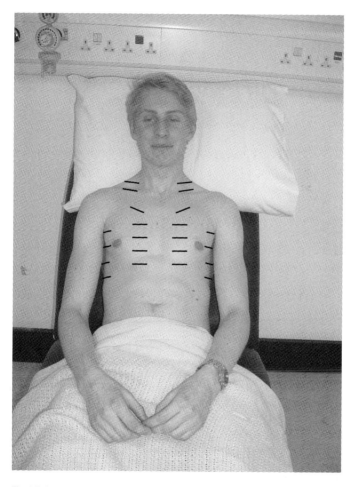

Fig 4.6 Anterior chest: zones for percussion and auscultation

- Whilst performing chest percussion, try to visualize the underlying anatomy. This will help with interpretation and diagnosis.
- Place the non-dominant hand on the patient's chest wall. The fingers should be slightly separated and the middle finger

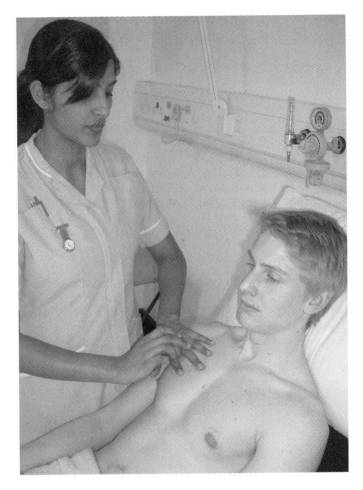

Fig 4.7 Chest percussion

should be pressed firmly into the intercostal space to be percussed (Ford *et al.*, 2005).

- Strike the centre of the middle phalanx of the middle finger sharply using the tip of the middle finger of the right hand (Ford *et al.*, 2005) (Figure 4.7). Deliver the stroke using a quick

Table 4.1 Percussion note abnormalities in respiratory disease

Major respiratory pathology	Percussion note abnormality
Normal chest	Normal percussion note
Pleural effusion	Stony dull to percussion (gravity dictates that this is at the lower part of the chest)
Pneumothorax	Hyper-resonant to percussion
COPD (emphysema)	Resonant to percussion
Lung fibrosis	Dull to percussion
Consolidation and collapse	Dull to percussion

COPD, chronic obstructive pulmonary disease.

flick of the wrist and finger joints, not from the arm or shoulder. The percussing finger should be bent so that its terminal phalanx is at right angles to the metacarpal bones when the blow is delivered and it strikes the percussed finger in a perpendicular manner. The percussing finger should then be removed immediately, like a clapper inside a bell, otherwise the resultant sound will be dampened (Epstein *et al.*, 2003).

- Percuss the anterior and lateral chest wall (Figure 4.6). Percuss from side to side, top to bottom, comparing both sides and looking for asymmetry.
- Categorize the percussion sounds (see Table 4.1).
- If an area of altered resonance is located, map out its boundaries by percussing from areas of normal to altered resonance (Ford *et al.*, 2005).
- Categorize the percussion sounds (see below).
- Record the findings and report as appropriate.

Chest auscultation

The diaphragm of the stethoscope (Figure 4.8) is used to auscultate the chest. The bell may be used for hairy chests. Expiration is normally quieter and shorter than inspiration, and there is no pause between the two. Normal breath sounds are only harsh near the trachea where noise is easily transmitted. Normal breath sounds are called vesicular sounds.

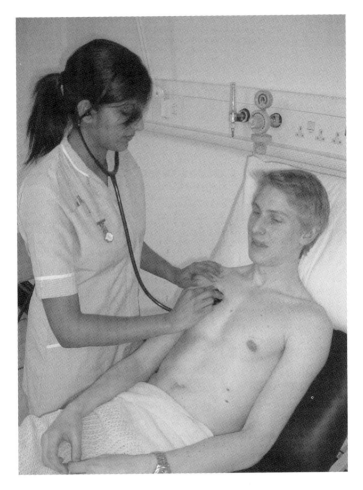

Fig 4.8 Chest auscultation

- Ask the patient to breathe in deeply through the nose and out through the mouth.
- Auscultate with the diaphragm in the three zones, in the apices and across the lateral chest on each side.

Box 4.3 Causes of lung collapse

- Consolidation of lung in pneumonia or distal to obstruction.
- Proximal endobronchial obstruction by tumour: can cause segmental, lobar or whole lung collapse.
- Retained secretions in patients with chronic obstructive pulmonary disease/bronchiectasis or in postoperative patients.
- Inhaled foreign bodies leading to proximal airway obstruction.

Table 4.2 Abnormalities of breath sounds on auscultation

Major respiratory pathology	Breath sound abnormality
Normal chest	Vesicular breathing
Pleural effusion	Reduced or absent breath sounds
Pneumothorax	Reduced or absent breath sounds
COPD (emphysema)	Reduced or absent breath sounds
Lung fibrosis	Reduced breath sounds
Consolidation and collapse	Bronchial breathing and whispering pectoriloquy

COPD, chronic obstructive pulmonary disease.

- Auscultate during inspiration and expiration. Decide whether the breath sounds are vesicular, bronchial, reduced or absent. Also note the area of lung affected and compare with palpation and percussion findings. If no breath sounds are heard over one side, this could indicate lung collapse (Box 4.3).

Bronchial breathing

Bronchial breathing involves abnormal breath sounds (Table 4.2) heard over consolidation or a collapsed lung, which conduct high frequencies well. The harsh breath sounds have a loud high-frequency component and are equal in inspiration and expiration, usually with a short gap between the two. Bronchial breathing can be imitated by listening over the trachea or larynx.

- Whispering high-pitched sounds, called whispering pectorilo-quy, accompany bronchial breathing when listening with the stethoscope.

Vocal resonance

Vocal resonance is the air carrying the voice produced in the larynx through the throat, mouth and nose (Marcovitch, 2005).

- Ask the patient to say quietly or whisper repeatedly the number '99'.
- Assess vocal resonance over the lung zones with a stethoscope, comparing both sides. Normally, high-pitched sounds are fil-tered out by healthy lung tissue; whispered sounds are heard to be loud over consolidated lung and areas of bronchial breathing. Diseases that cause reduced or absent breath sounds will also cause reduced vocal resonance.

Tactile vocal fremitus

Tactile vocal fremitus is palpation of the vibration caused by vocal resonance. It is not routinely undertaken as it duplicates the findings of vocal resonance assessment. However, tactile vocal fremitus is observed over consolidated lung, and can add to the findings.

Added sounds

The chest can be auscultated for added sounds, e.g. crackles, wheeze, stridor and pleural rub (the terms 'rhonchi', 'rales' and 'crepitations' have been replaced by the simpler terms 'crackles' and 'wheeze'):

- *Crackles*: described as fine or coarse; fine crackles (often described as the sound made when walking gently on virgin snow) can be heard at the end of inspiration in lung fibrosis and pulmonary oedema; coarse crackles (often described as the sound made by breakfast cereal in milk) can be heard in inspiration and expiration over areas of bronchiectasis and consolidation. Crackles represent the opening and closing of bronchioles.

- *Wheeze*: normally polyphonic (different pitches) and heard in expiration; it represents the limitation of flow in different sized medium and small airways. Wheeze is widespread in asthma and can be heard in exacerbations of COPD. Wheeze can be monophonic (a single pitch) if a tumour obstructs a large airway and is localized to a single area of the chest.

- *Stridor*: inspiratory noise (Cox & Roper, 2005) louder than wheeze and often heard as a groan or a crowing, representing large, partial upper airway obstruction, e.g. foreign body, laryngeal oedema. It is usually accompanied by a high respiratory rate and respiratory distress. An ear, nose and throat emergency, it requires urgent and careful attention.

- *Pleural rub*: a creaking or rubbing sound heard in a localized area with the stethoscope. It represents inflammation or thickening of the pleura, which normally slide gently over each other during breathing (Douglas *et al.*, 2005).

Examination of the posterior aspect of the chest

Examination of the posterior aspect of the chest is very similar to that of the anterior aspect, which has been described above. The three zones for percussion and auscultation are detailed in Figure 4.9. There is no cardiac dullness at the back, and percussion and auscultation of the lower zones can reveal pathology not encountered anteriorly. Use the three zones to guide the examination and repeat palpation for chest expansion, percussion and auscultation at the back.

For percussion:

- Sit the patient forward and percuss the posterior chest wall, omitting the areas covered by the scapulae (Figure 4.10). Ask the patient to move the elbows forward across the front of the chest: this will rotate the scapulae anteriorly and out of the way (Talley & O'Connor, 2001). It may be helpful to offer the patient a pillow to lean on (Bickle *et al.*, 2002). Again percuss

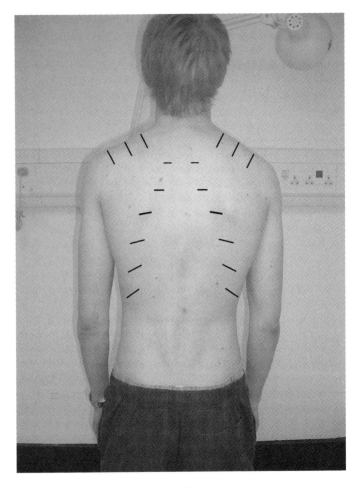

Fig 4.9 Posterior chest: zones for percussion and auscultation

from side to side, top to bottom, comparing both sides and looking for asymmetry. Do not forget that the lung extends much further down posteriorly than anteriorly (Epstein *et al.*, 2003).

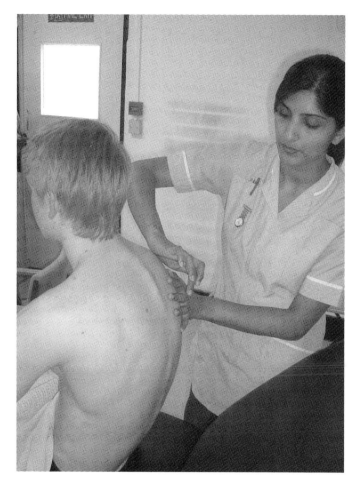

Fig 4.10 Posterior chest: chest percussion

Additional information

Further clues to the underlying diagnosis may be available at the bedside. A peak flow meter can often be found and a bedside peak expiratory flow rate measurement can be taken at the end of the examination. The patient's temperature and oxygen saturation are recorded on the observations chart and should be noted.

CONCLUSION

Examination of the respiratory system should follow a methodical approach to ensure that important signs and symptoms are not missed. The importance of respiratory history, peripheral examination of the respiratory system and chest examination has been described in this chapter.

REFERENCES

Bickle I, Hamilton P, McClusky D, Kelly B (2002) *Clinical Skills for Medical Students: a Hands-On Guide*. PasTest Ltd., Knutsford, Cheshire.

Cox N & Roper T (2005) *Clinical Skills: Oxford Core Text*. Oxford University Press, Oxford.

Douglas G, Nicol F, Robertson C (2005) *MacLeod's Clinical Examination*, 11th edn. Elsevier, Edinburgh.

Epstein O, Perkin G, Cookson J, de Bono D (2003) *Clinical Examination*, 3rd edn. Mosby, London.

Ford M, Hennessey I, Japp A (2005) *Introduction to Clinical Examination*. Elsevier, Oxford.

Gleadle J (2004) *History and Examination at a Glance*. Blackwell Publishing, Oxford.

Marcovitch H (2005) *Black's Medical Dictionary*, 41st edn. A & C Black, London.

McFerran T, Martin E (2003) *Mini-Dictionary for Nurses*, 5th edn. Oxford University Press, Oxford.

Talley N, O'Connor S (2001) *Clinical Examination: a Systematic Guide to Physical Diagnosis*. Blackwell Science, Oxford.

Thomas J, Monaghan T (2007) *Oxford Handbook of Clinical Examination and Practical Skills*. Oxford University Press, Oxford.

Ward J, Leach R, Wiener C (2006) *The Respiratory System at a Glance*, 2nd edn. Blackwell Publishing, Oxford.

Examination of the Gastrointestinal and Genitourinary Systems

5

Yi-Yang Ng

INTRODUCTION

Examination of the gastrointestinal and genitourinary systems includes the gastrointestinal tract from mouth to anus and the organs within the abdominal cavity, as well as the groins, external genitalia, digital rectal examination and vaginal examination (if appropriate). Examination should follow a systematic approach: inspection, palpation, percussion and auscultation.

The aim of this chapter is to provide an understanding of the examination of the gastrointestinal and genitourinary systems.

LEARNING OUTCOMES

At the end of this chapter, the reader will be able to:

❏ List the symptoms of gastrointestinal disease.
❏ Describe the peripheral examination of the gastrointestinal system.
❏ Describe the examination of the abdomen.
❏ Discuss the examination of the groins and hernial orifices.
❏ List the symptoms of genitourinary disease.
❏ Outline the examination of the male and female genitalia.
❏ Describe digital examination of the rectum.

SYMPTOMS OF GASTROINTESTINAL DISEASE

Symptoms of gastrointestinal disease include:

• Dysphagia.
• Heartburn.

- Nausea.
- Vomiting.
- Diarrhoea.
- Abdominal pain.
- Mass.
- Rectal bleeding.
- Change in bowel habit.
- Anorexia/weight loss.
- Jaundice.

(Sources: Gleadle, 2004; Ford *et al.*, 2005)

PERIPHERAL EXAMINATION OF THE GASTROINTESTINAL SYSTEM

Peripheral examination of the gastrointestinal system should follow a methodical approach:

- Look at the patient and note any signs of malnutrition, dehydration (tongue and skin turgor) and jaundice (Ford *et al.*, 2005).
- Examine the patient's fingernails: observe for leuconychia (white discoloration of the fingernails caused by low albumin or chronic ill health), koilonychia (spooning or concave appearance of the nail caused by severe iron deficiency) and clubbing (sometimes caused by cirrhosis, inflammatory bowel disease or coeliac disease) (Thomas & Monaghan, 2007).
- Check for asterixis: same as that which can be observed in hypercapnia (see pp. 81–82); characteristic of encephalopathy caused by hepatic failure.
- Check the upper limbs, face, neck and upper chest for spider naevi (a sign of chronic liver disease) (Marcovitch, 2005).
- Gently retract the lower eyelid: observe the conjunctiva for pallor (a sign of anaemia) and the scelera for jaundice (Ford *et al.*, 2005).
- Check the mouth for evidence of thrush or ulcers.
- Examine the tongue: look for glossitis (smooth red swelling of the tongue); causes include deficiency in iron, vitamin B12 or folate (Thomas & Monaghan, 2007).

- Palpate the supraclavicular region: check for lymph nodes.
- Examine the male breasts: gynaecomastia can be associated with liver disease (Ford *et al.*, 2005).

EXAMINATION OF THE ABDOMEN

Surface anatomy of the abdomen

The abdomen can be divided into nine distinctive regions by two imaginary vertical lines and horizontal lines (Lumley, 2002) (Figure 5.1). The vertical lines run between the mid-clavicular point and mid-inguinal point on each side. The upper horizontal line is also known as the subcostal plane because it crosses the tips of the costal margins. The lower horizontal line crosses the upper border of the iliac crests and is known as the transtubercular line.

Inspection of the abdomen

- Lie the patient supine on one pillow with both arms by the sides (some patients with breathing difficulties or problems with the thoracic spine may need more than one pillow).
- Make sure the patient is comfortable before proceeding.
- Expose the patient from the nipples to the pubic symphysis. The external genitalia can be exposed for assessment later, if indicated.
- Stand at the end of the bed and note the shape of the abdomen, movement of the abdomen with respiration, symmetry of the abdomen, obvious mass, scar and stoma.
- Look for general surgery-related scars on the abdomen (Box 5.1).

General palpation of the abdomen

- Approach from the right-hand side of the patient.
- Adopt a position such that the examining hand is at the same level as the patient.
- Ask the patient if there is any pain or discomfort in the abdomen; if there is, palpate this area last.

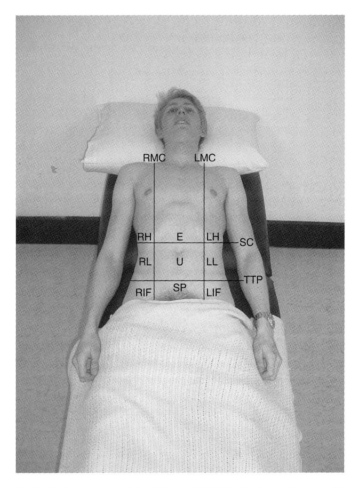

Fig 5.1 Surface anatomy of the abdomen. RIF, Right iliac fossa; SP, suprapubic region; LIF, left iliac fossa, RH, right hypochondrial region; E, Epigastric region, LH, left hypochondrial region; SL, Subcostal plane; RL, right lumbar region; U, umbilical region; LL, left lumbar region; TTP, transtubercular plane; LMC, left midclavular line; RMC, right midclavular line

Box 5.1 Surgery-related scars

- Long mid-line scar, e.g. previous laparotomy.
- Right subcostal scar (Kocher's incision), e.g. previous open cholecystectomy.
- Grid-iron incison scar, e.g. previous appendicectomy.
- Transverse suprapubic incision (Pfannenstiel) scar, e.g. previous pelvic surgery.

(Source: Lumley, 2002)

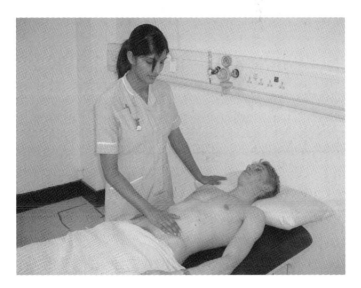

Fig 5.2 Light palpation of the abdomen

- Perform light palpation by gently pressing the patient's abdomen using the flat of the hand (Figure 5.2) throughout the nine regions (Figure 5.1), whilst watching the patient's face for any sign of discomfort, e.g. grimace. The purpose of light palpation is to check for tenderness, guarding, rebound tenderness and rigidity.

Box 5.2 Possible causes of palpable abdominal mass arising from each region of the abdomen

- *Left hypochondrium*: spleen, splenic flexure of the colon.
- *Right hypochondrium*: liver, hepatic flexure of the colon, gall bladder.
- *Epigastrium*: stomach, duodenum, pancreas, transverse colon.
- *Left lumbar region*: descending colon, left kidney.
- *Right lumbar region*: ascending colon, right kidney.
- *Umbilical region*: abdominal aorta, small bowel.
- *Left iliac fossa*: sigmoid colon, left ovary.
- *Right iliac fossa*: caecum, appendix, right ovary.
- *Suprapubic region*: urinary bladder, uterus.

- Perform deep palpation by pressing each of the nine regions deeper. This technique can be performed using one hand or both hands with one on top of the other.
- The purpose of deep palpation is to detect any abnormal mass and its characteristics. Possible causes of palpable abdominal mass are listed in Box 5.2.

Signs of peritonitis

Guarding: involuntary abdominal musculature contraction over an inflamed organ and peritoneum.

Rebound tenderness: pain on removal of pressure rather than application of pressure to the abdomen.

Rigidity: extension of guarding which involves the entire abdominal musculature.

Palpation of enlarged abdominal organs
Liver
Normally, the lower edge of the liver is not palpable, and it is not possible to palpate the upper edge of the liver as it normally lies within the rib cage. The liver enlarges inferior from the right costal margin in the direction of the right iliac fossa and moves inferiorly during inspiration.

Procedure for palpation of the liver

- Place the radial aspect of the index finger over the patient's right iliac fossa and ask the patient to breathe in and out as instructed (Figure 5.3).

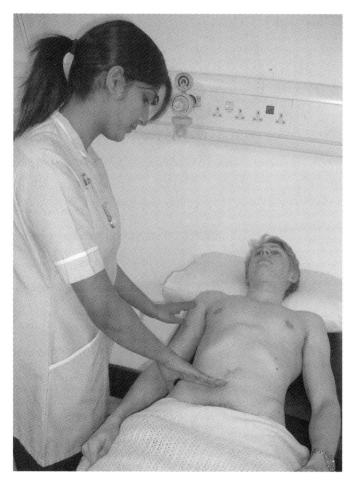

Fig 5.3 Palpation of the liver

- During inspiration, move the finger towards the right costal margin and, during expiration, hold the finger steady.
- Work up towards the right costal margin with each breath until the edge of the liver hits the finger.
- If the lower edge of the liver is palpable, note the surface and edge, its shape, size (in centimetres below the right costal margin), texture, tenderness and pulsatility.

Spleen

Normally, the spleen is not palpable. It enlarges inferiorly and medially towards the right iliac fossa and descends during inspiration.

Procedure for palpation of the spleen

- Start by asking the patient to turn slightly on to the right side and place the non-examining hand on the patient's left lower ribs from behind. This manoeuvre splints the lower ribs, making the spleen easier to palpate anteriorly.
- Place the radial aspect of the index finger over the patient's right iliac fossa and ask the patient to breathe in and out as instructed.
- During inspiration, move the finger towards the left costal margin and, during expiration, hold the finger steady (Figure 5.4).
- Work up towards the left costal margin with each breath until the edge of the spleen hits the finger.

Kidneys

The kidneys are retroperitoneal structures that do not move with respiration. Palpation of the kidneys requires a bimanual technique.

Procedure for palpation of the kidneys

- Lie the patient supine, and place the left hand behind the flank and the right hand just beneath the costal margin at the lumbar region.

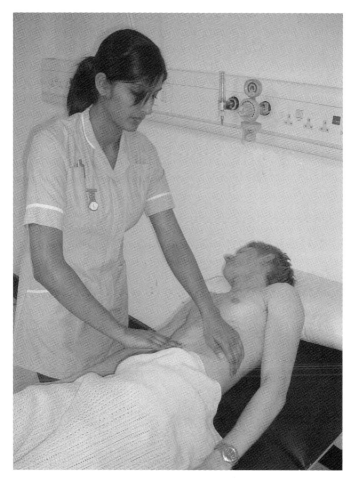

Fig 5.4 Palpation of the spleen

- Flip the kidney up from below, and palpate for the kidney using the other hand (Figure 5.5). This is also known as 'balloting' the kidney (Douglas *et al.*, 2005).
- Repeat the same procedure on the other kidney.

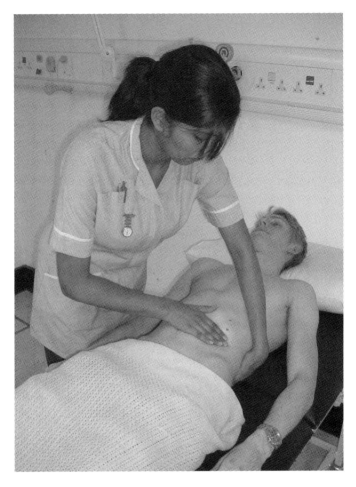

Fig 5.5 Bimanual technique for palpation of the kidney

Differentiation of an enlarged spleen from an enlarged left kidney on palpation

Sometimes, it can be difficult to differentiate an enlarged left kidney from an enlarged spleen; the following features may help to resolve this matter (Talley & O'Connor, 2006):

- The spleen enlarges diagonally in the direction of the right iliac fossa.
- The spleen is dull to percussion, whereas there is resonance over the kidney.
- It is not possible to get on top of the spleen.

Aorta

The abdominal aorta bifurcates at the level of the umbilicus. In a thin patient, pulsation may be felt in the abdomen; if the fingers are displaced to the sides, this is known as expansile pulsation, and is suggestive of an abdominal aortic aneurysm (Cox & Roper, 2005).

Procedure for palpation of an abdominal aortic aneurysm

- Place the flat of the hand at the mid-line above the umbilicus and press down firmly.
- If pulsation is felt, place the index fingers on either side of the pulsation and observe whether the fingers move apart with each pulsation, suggesting an abdominal aortic aneurysm.

Urinary bladder

The urinary bladder is a pelvic organ and is not normally palpable. In the presence of urinary retention, the urinary bladder can rise up to the level of the umbilicus (Talley & O'Connor, 2006).

Procedure for palpation of the urinary bladder

- Use the flat of the right hand and start to palpate from the umbilical region, moving towards the suprapubic region, until the edge of the urinary bladder is reached.
- Characteristically, it is not possible to locate the base of the urinary bladder, and it can be tender (or uncomfortable) with dullness to percussion in the presence of an excessive amount of urine in urinary retention.
- In females, an enlarged uterus can sometimes be mistaken for the urinary bladder; imaging investigations may be indicated.

Percussion of the abdomen

Percussion is normally performed by placing the left middle finger firmly on the skin, which is struck by the middle finger of the right hand using a series of two blows at each position. The blows should be delivered by bending the wrist. Percussion over a hollow organ, such as the bowel, generates a resonant note; percussion over a solid structure or fluid generates a dull note (Urbano & Fedorowski, 2000).

Liver

In a normal abdomen, it is not possible to percuss the lower edge of the liver. Percussion over the liver produces a dull note.

Procedure for percussion of the liver

- Percuss from the right iliac fossa to the right hypochondrium for the lower edge of the liver (Figure 5.6).
- If the lower edge of the liver is detected in the abdomen (dull note to percussion), percuss to determine the position of the upper border of the liver (to differentiate whether the liver is enlarged or displaced inferiorly by respiratory disease): percuss from the right mid-clavicular region to the right costal margin. The upper border of the liver is normally in the right fifth intercostal space.

Spleen

In a normal abdomen, it is not possible to percuss the lower edge of the spleen. Percussion over the spleen produces a dull note.

Procedure for percussion of the spleen

- Percuss from the right iliac fossa to the left hypochondrium for the lower edge of the spleen (Figure 5.7).

Ascites

Ascites is defined as the presence of fluid in the peritoneal cavity. In the presence of abdominal distension, it is important to make sure that ascites is not overlooked.

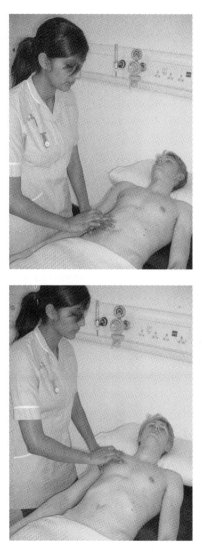

Fig 5.6 Abdominal percussion: the liver

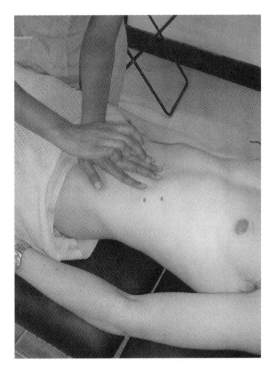

Fig 5.7 Abdominal percussion: the spleen

Procedure to detect mild to moderate ascites:
shifting dullness

- Percuss from the mid-line to the left flank until the percussion note changes from tympanitic to dull.
- Roll the patient to the right (towards you) and wait for 30 s for the fluid to redistribute.
- Percuss again; the percussion note in the left flank changes from dull to tympanitic as a result of the redistribution of fluid.
- Percuss from the flank back to the mid-line; the percussion note in the mid-line should become dull. If the dullness has shifted, the test is positive for ascites (shifting dullness).

Procedure to detect massive ascites: fluid thrill

- Remember to warn the patient prior to this procedure.
- Ask the patient to put one hand (ulnar aspect) on the abdomen. The purpose of this is to prevent the movement of fat which may feel like a thrill (Douglas *et al.*, 2005).
- Place the left hand on the patient's left flank and flick the abdomen on the other side. A thrill is felt as a result of movement of fluid.

Auscultation of the abdomen
Using the diaphragm of the stethoscope, the abdomen should be auscultated for bowel sounds and to exclude any vascular bruits.

Procedure for auscultation of bowel sounds and vascular bruits

- Place the stethoscope on the abdomen (it does not matter where the stethoscope is placed) and listen for bowel sounds (Box 5.3) for at least 1 min.
- Place the stethoscope above the umbilicus for abdominal aortic bruits.
- Place the stethoscope 2 cm lateral to the umbilicus on both sides for renal bruits.

EXAMINATION OF THE GROINS AND HERNIAL ORIFICES
This is an important part of the abdominal examination, especially in a patient presenting with groin hernia and other groin swelling. This is a very sensitive part of the human body and it is important to be especially gentle whilst examining this area.

Box 5.3 Types of bowel sound
- Normal: gurgling every 10–20 s.
- Borborygmi: increased activity.
- High pitched and tinkling: intestinal obstruction.
- Absent: paralytic ileus.

Surface anatomy of the groin

It is important to understand the surface anatomy of the groin. The bony landmarks important to this context are the pubic symphysis, pubic tubercles and the anterior superior iliac spines. The inguinal ligament runs between the anterior superior iliac spine and the pubic tubercle.

The inguinal canal, a tube-like structure situated just above the medial half of the inguinal ligament, consists of two openings: the deep ring and superficial ring. The deep ring is located at the mid-point between the anterior superior iliac spine and pubic tubercle; this is known as the mid-point of the inguinal ligament. The superficial ring is located above and medial to the pubic tubercle. The mid-inguinal point is situated at the mid-point between the anterior superior iliac spine and the pubic symphysis (Lumley, 2002).

Procedure for examination of the groins and hernial orifices

- With the patient standing up, expose the groin and external genitalia.
- Ask the patient to produce a strong cough, whilst observing the groin; if a visible cough impulse (i.e. presence of a swelling during coughing) is detected, place the hand over the swelling and check whether there is a palpable cough impulse.
- Assess the inguinal swelling in relation to the inguinal ligament and pubic tubercle. Differences in groin herniae are detailed in Table 5.1.
- Ask the patient to try to reduce the hernia.
- If the hernia is reducible, place the fingers over the deep ring and check whether the hernia is controlled by this pressure or reappears on coughing.
- Proceed with examination of the remainder of the groin and the external genitalia.

Table 5.1 Differences in groin herniae on clinical examination

	Types of groin hernia		
	Indirect inguinal hernia	**Direct inguinal hernia**	**Femoral hernia**
Origin	Above the inguinal ligament	Above the inguinal ligament	Beneath the inguinal ligament
Relation to pubic tubercle	Above	Above	Below
Scrotal extension	Extends into the scrotum	Rarely extends into the scrotum	Never extends into the scrotum
Reducibility	Reducible	Reducible	Rarely reducible
Cough impulse	Present	Present	Rarely present
Controlled by deep ring pressure	Yes	No	No

Other conditions that may present as groin swellings

If the groin swelling does not appear to be a groin hernia, consider the possibility of the following conditions:

- Enlarged groin lymph node.
- Saphena varix.
- Ectopic testicle.
- Psoas abscess.
- Lipoma.

(Browse *et al.*, 2005)

SYMPTOMS OF GENITOURINARY DISEASE

The symptoms of genitourinary disease include:

- Dysuria/urgency.
- Haematuria.
- Urinary frequency.
- Nocturia.
- Urinary incontinence.
- Menstrual cycle irregularities.

- Sexual dysfunction.
- Urethral/vaginal discharge.

(Sources: Gleadle, 2004; Ford *et al.*, 2005)

EXAMINATION OF THE MALE AND FEMALE GENITALIA

This is a very sensitive part of the human body and it is important to be very gentle whilst assessing this area and to ensure that a chaperone is present. It is important to remember to wear gloves.

Procedure for examination of the male external genitalia

- Either leave the patient in a standing position (following groin assessment) or ask him to lie flat on the couch.
- Inspect the patient's pubic hair distribution and scrotum, groin crease and penis for rash, swelling or infestation.
- Palpate each scrotum individually for scrotal skin swelling.
- Palpate each testicle in turn between forefinger and thumb, and compare the sizes of both testicles.
- Palpate the epididymis and spermatic cord on each side. If it is possible to palpate above the swelling within the scrotum, it is not an inguinal hernia.
- Transilluminate any scrotal swelling using a pen-torch to identify its nature; a cystic structure glows.

Procedure for examination of the female external genitalia

Because of its intimate nature, vaginal examination should be performed by trained personnel following informed consent, and a chaperone should be present throughout the examination.

- Position the patient either on her back with the hips and knees flexed and thighs apart or in the left lateral position.
- Ensure adequate lighting and don a pair of gloves before proceeding.
- Separate the labia majora using the left index and middle fingers and inspect the clitoris, urethra, vagina and any abnormality of the vaginal wall.

- Ask the patient to cough and/or strain down: note whether vaginal wall prolapse or urinary incontinence occurs.

Vaginal examination

- Inform the patient that you are about to insert two fingers into her vagina in order to feel the uterus (womb).
- Apply lubricating gel to your right index and middle fingers and insert the examining fingers gently and slowly.
- Feel the cervix with the tips of your fingers.
- Place the examining fingers at the anterior fornix of the vagina and press the lower abdomen of the patient with the left hand. Try to feel the uterus between the two hands; check size, shape, mobility and tenderness.
- Inform the patient when withdrawing the fingers (gently and slowly).
- Wipe away the lubricating gel from the patient with tissue paper.

DIGITAL EXAMINATION OF THE RECTUM

Explain to the patient and obtain consent prior to the procedure. It is important to let the patient know in advance that the examination may be uncomfortable, but pain is rarely felt if performed appropriately. Assemble the necessary equipment: a pair of non-sterile gloves, lubricating gel and tissue paper for cleaning up following the procedure.

Procedure

- Ensure that there is adequate lighting throughout the procedure.
- Position the patient in the left lateral position with the knees resting close to the chest and the buttocks at the edge of the couch; expose the buttocks.
- Don a pair of gloves and separate the buttocks.
- Inspect the perineum, anus and perianal area for skin tags, anal fissure, fistula-in-ano, anal warts and external piles.

- Apply some lubricating gel to the right index finger and begin palpation by pressing the finger against the anal verge and gently advancing the gloved finger into the rectum.
- Palpate the anterior, posterior and lateral parts of the rectum by turning the wrist.
- Anteriorly, feel for the prostate gland in the male and the cervix in the female.
- Before withdrawing the finger, ask the patient to 'squeeze' the finger to check for anal tone (Douglas *et al.*, 2005).
- On withdrawal, check the gloved finger for blood, mucus or pus, melaena and colour of the stool.
- Clean the patient's perineum and help the patient to get dressed.

CONCLUSION

Examination of the gastrointestinal system should follow a systematic approach: inspection, palpation, percussion and auscultation. In this chapter, the taking of a gastrointestinal history, peripheral examination of the gastrointestinal system, examination of the abdomen and examination of the groins have been described. Examination of the male and female genitalia and digital examination of the rectum have been outlined.

REFERENCES

Browse N, Black J, Burnand K, Thomas W (2005) *Browse's Introduction to the Symptoms and Signs of Surgical Diseases*, 4th edn. Hodder Education, London.

Cox N, Roper T (2005) *Clinical Skills: Oxford Core Text*. Oxford University Press, Oxford.

Douglas G, Nicol F, Robertson C (2005) *MacLeod's Clinical Examination*, 11th edn. Elsevier, Edinburgh.

Ford M, Hennessey I, Japp A (2005) *Introduction to Clinical Examination*. Elsevier, Oxford.

Gleadle J (2004) *History and Examination at a Glance*. Blackwell Publishing, Oxford.

Lumley J (2002) *Surface Anatomy: the Anatomical Basis of Clinical Examination*, 3rd edn. Churchill Livingstone, Edinburgh.

Marcovitch H (2005) *Black's Medical Dictionary*, 41st edn. A & C Black, London.

Talley N, O'Connor S (2006) *Clinical Examination: a Systematic Guide to Physical Diagnosis*, 5th edn. Elsevier, Edinburgh.

Thomas J, Monaghan T (2007) *Oxford Handbook of Clinical Examination and Practical Skills*. Oxford University Press, Oxford.

Urbano F, Fedorowski J (2000) Review of clinical signs: medical percussion. *Hospital Physician* **9**: 31–36.

Examination of the Neurological System

6

Gareth Walters

INTRODUCTION

Although the examination of the neurological system fills some practitioners with a sense of dread, it is actually one of the easiest examinations to perform and has the added benefit that all the signs elicited are very obvious (Cox & Roper, 2005). The examination should include an assessment of the conscious level and an examination of the cranial nerves, limbs and cerebellum. As with the examination of other systems, a methodical approach is essential.

The aim of this chapter is to provide an understanding of the examination of the neurological system.

LEARNING OUTCOMES

At the end of this chapter, the reader will be able to

❏ List the symptoms of neurological disease.
❏ Describe the assessment of the conscious level.
❏ Outline the examination of the cranial nerves.
❏ Discuss the examination of the lower limbs.
❏ Discuss the examination of the upper limbs.
❏ Outline the examination of the cerebellum.

SYMPTOMS OF NEUROLOGICAL DISEASE

The symptoms of neurological disease include:

- Headaches.
- Fits.
- Blackouts.
- Collapses.

- Falls.
- Weaknesses.
- Unsteadiness.
- Tremor.
- Visual, hearing and sensory disorders.

(Sources: Gleadle, 2004; Ford *et al.*, 2005)

ASSESSMENT OF THE CONSCIOUS LEVEL

The conscious level refers to the awareness of patients of their surroundings and their responsiveness to certain stimuli, such as pain or verbal commands. Causes of altered conscious level include compression or damage to the brainstem, intracranial disease and diffuse brain dysfunction.

The assessment of the conscious level is useful in a variety of clinical situations including:

- Attempting to establish whether a patient is acutely ill.
- Determining whether the airway is at risk of being compromised.
- Measuring improvement in the patient's condition.
- Evaluating the response to treatment.
- Gauging the prognosis in critically ill patients.
- Determining the degree of recovery following general anaesthesia or sedation.

Patients can be classified according to conscious level, and the two most commonly used systems for classification are the Glasgow Coma Scale and the AVPU scale.

Glasgow Coma Scale

The Glasgow Coma Scale (GCS) is a 15-point scale described by Jennet and Teasdale (1974). The evaluation of the conscious level involves the scoring of the response in three areas: eye opening, verbal response and motor response (Box 6.1). It was intended for use with patients with head injuries as an initial assessment of severity, and as a predictor of complications. It is accurate in predicting a deterioration in condition and is now widely used

---

Box 6.1 Glasgow Coma Scale (GCS)

Score (total out of 15).

Eye opening (E):

- Spontaneous   4
- To speech   3
- To pain   2
- None   1

Verbal response (V):

- Orientated   5
- Confused conversation   4
- Inappropriate words   3
- Incomprehensible words 2
- None   1

Best motor response (M):

- Obeys commands   6
- Localizes pain   5
- Normal flexion (withdrawal)   4
- Abnormal flexion (decorticate)   3
- Extension (decerebrate)   2
- None   1

[Adapted from the National Institute for
Clinical Excellence (NICE) 2007]

---

in the assessment of the conscious level. The National Institute
for Clinical Excellence (NICE) guidelines for head injuries (NICE,
2007) recommend that all patients with a head injury should have
a GCS score measured on arrival at hospital. Patients with a GCS
score of less than 15 should be assessed immediately by trained
staff.

A GCS score of 9 out of 15 is defined as coma (NICE, 2007), and
indicates the need to protect the patient's airway from aspiration
or asphyxiation. In a head injury, a GCS score of 14 implies a mild
head injury, 9–13 moderate and less than 9 severe.

1 Assessment of 'eye opening'.
   - Introduce yourself and ask the patient 'can you hear me?' or 'open your eyes!'. If the patient's eyes are open, a score of 4 is given for 'spontaneous' eye opening. If the patient opens the eyes only when asked, this responds 'to speech'.
   - If there is no response to speech, assess the response to pain by applying a painful stimulus, e.g. press on the supraorbital ridge or squeeze the little finger (Figure 6.1).
   - Score 'eye opening' according to the GCS (Box 6.1).
2 Assessment of the best 'verbal response'.
   - Assess the patient's verbal response by talking and asking questions. Establish whether the patient is orientated or confused. It may be necessary to evaluate the patient's verbal response following a painful stimulus.
   - Score the best 'verbal response' according to the GCS (Box 6.1).
3 Assessment of the best 'motor response'.
   - Observe the patient for purposeful spontaneous movement in the upper limbs (spinal reflexes can cause spontaneous movement in the lower limbs that are not purposeful).
   - If there is no spontaneous movement, ask the patient to 'squeeze my fingers' and note whether there is a purposeful response.
   - Again, if there is no spontaneous movement, apply a painful stimulus. Look carefully at the categories. If the patient moves towards the painful stimulus, this represents localization to pain; if the patient moves away, this represents withdrawal from pain. As the conscious level deteriorates, motor function deteriorates and the patient exhibits abnormal flexion (decorticate – contraction of the flexors of the upper limbs bilaterally) or abnormal extension (decerebrate – contraction of the extensors of the upper and lower limbs bilaterally).
   - Note the GCS score on the neurological observation chart alongside the respiratory rate, pupil sizes and responses, temperature, blood pressure and heart rate. Any lateralizing

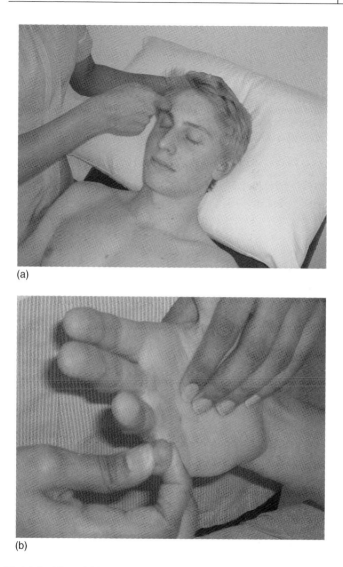

(a)

(b)

Fig 6.1 Applying painful stimuli: supraorbital ridge pressure (a) and little finger pressure (b)

Table 6.1 AVPU scale (Source: Resuscitation Council UK, 2006)

Score	Rationale
Alert	Fully awake (although not necessarily orientated) and with spontaneous movement
Responds to voice (Voice)	The patient makes any response when talked to, which could be in any of the three components: Eyes, Voice or Motor
Responds to pain (Pain)	The patient makes a response in any of the three component measures when a pain stimulus is used
Unresponsive	Also seen noted as 'Unconscious'; no Eye, Voice or Motor response to voice or pain

weakness (lack of movement of one side or limb) should also be noted.

AVPU scale

The AVPU scale (Table 6.1) is a recommended tool to quickly and effectively assess the level of consciousness in a critically ill patient (Resuscitation Council UK, 2006). It is incorporated into many 'Early Warning Score' systems for critically ill patients, as it is a simpler tool than GCS. It is not suitable for long-term neurological observation. Mackay *et al.* (2000) found that 'Responds to voice' correlates with a GCS score of 13, and the division between 'Responds to voice' and 'Responds to pain' correlates with a GCS score of 9.

EXAMINATION OF THE CRANIAL NERVES

This examination looks at the 12 cranial nerves (I–XII). The abnormal signs are striking and show obvious deviation from the routine. It is helpful to understand the common cranial nerve defects.

There are many variations on a theme, but a simple, minute-long routine that can easily be reproduced using the minimum of equipment (e.g. a pen-torch) is preferable and practical. The routine is a screen for cranial nerve problems; further tests can be performed if a problem is identified.

Before undertaking the examination, it is important to sit opposite the patient on the same eye level and to observe for any obvious abnormalities in facial expression. If appropriate, ask patients to wear their spectacles.

Examination of the olfactory nerve (I)

- Check the patency of both nostrils by asking the patient to sniff; anosmia (loss of sense of smell) is usually caused by nasal disease (Ford *et al.*, 2005).
- Ask the patient if there has been any change in smell.
- Ask the patient to close the eyes and to identify a common odour, e.g. orange peel; this is subtle and can discriminate any problems with smell.

Examination of the optic nerve (II)
Visual acuity

- Test the visual acuity of each eye separately.
- Ask the patient to cover one eye with the hand; show your hand and ask how many fingers are being held up (Figure 6.2).
- If the patient cannot see the fingers, the visual acuity is very poor: ask whether the hand or, indeed, the torchlight can be seen.
- Once both eyes have been tested, discern differences in acuity between them.
- Use a Snellen chart (Figure 6.3) if formal measurement of visual acuity is required; use Ishihara plates if colour vision requires testing.
- Examine the pupils (II, afferent; III, efferent) and establish pupil size, reaction to light and accommodation.
- Ask the patient to 'look straight ahead' and observe the pupil size in normal light; normal, constricted or dilated will suffice, although many neurological observation charts specify a pupil size on a scale of 1–5.

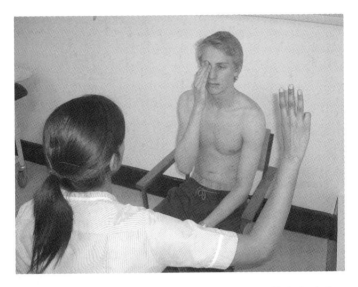

Fig 6.2 Testing visual acuity: ask the patient to cover one eye with the hand; show your hand and ask how many fingers are being held up

Visual fields

- Sit facing the patient, a metre away, with the eyes at roughly the same level as the patient's eyes; maintain eye-to-eye contact.
- Cover your left eye with the left hand and ask the patient to cover his/her right eye with the right hand.
- Ask the patient to look directly at your nose and to say when your fingers can be seen; with your right hand equidistant between yourself and the patient, bring two fingers in diagonally towards the mid-line. It is possible to judge whether the patient sees the fingers at the same time as you in the peripheral visual fields. Test the four quadrants (Figure 6.4) and repeat the above procedures with the other eye.

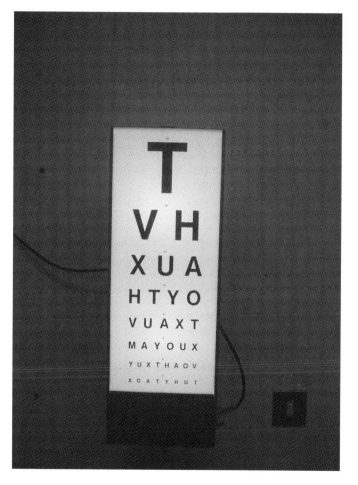

Fig 6.3 A Snellen chart: for formal measurement of visual acuity

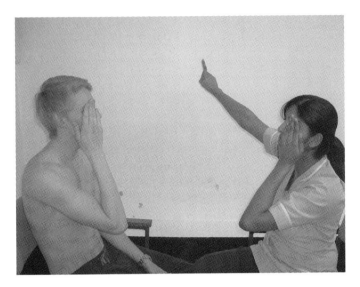

Fig 6.4 Testing the visual fields: test the four quadrants

Examination of the oculomotor, trochlear and abducens nerves (III, IV, VI)
Pupillary reflexes

- In a darkened room, move a torchlight towards the pupil from the side to the patient's face and observe any change in pupil size. The pupil should constrict when exposed to direct light (direct light reflex). Take care not to shine the light in the other eye, but note whether the opposite pupil also constricts (consensual reflex). Repeat this manoeuvre on the other eye. Lesions of nerves II or III will produce deficits in direct and consensual reflexes.
- Assess accommodation in both pupils.
- Position the finger at least 1 m from the patient and ask the patient to focus on it.
- Ask the patient to follow the finger as it is moved within 20 cm of the nose.

- Observe both eyes for the pupillary changes of accommodation. When refocusing from a distant to a near image, both eyes should converge and the pupils should constrict. Efferent (III) or afferent (II) nerve lesions produce deficits in constriction.
- Observe for central visual field defects by using a red hat-pin (or a red neuro-tip). Repeat the procedure, but move the object around the central tunnel of vision rather than throughout the peripheral fields (the patient needs to be able to recognize that the object is red). Position the object directly in front of the eye and ask the patient if it can be seen and, if so, what is its colour. Then proceed to check the central fields, reminding the patient to say whether the pin disappears or whether it does not appear to be red anymore; this is to detect central scotoma of visual loss – red is the first component of central vision to be lost.

Ocular movements

- Assess ocular movements. Sit directly in front of the patient and hold up an index finger. Ask the patient whether the finger can be seen and, if so, whether it appears 'double': the presence of diplopia (double vision) at rest indicates an extraocular muscle problem.
- If there is no double vision, ask the patient to keep the head still and to follow your finger with the eyes as it is moved away; the development of blurred vision again indicates a more subtle extraocular muscle problem caused by eye movement.
- Ensure that the patient's eyes are entrained to extremes of gaze and look for lack of movement. Ensure that all extraocular muscle gazes are tested (see Figure 6.5). Also look for nystagmus (jerking eye movements) at the extremes of lateral gaze.

Examination of the trigeminal and facial nerves (V, VII)
Sensory function (V)

- Assess the corneal reflex (often the first trigeminal nerve function to disappear).

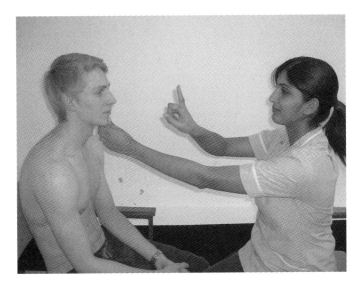

Fig 6.5 Testing all extraocular muscle gazes

- Roll up a piece of cotton wool or tissue paper and ask the patient to turn to the left.
- After warning the patient that it may be uncomfortable and may make him/her blink, touch the corner of the eye (see Figure 6.6).
- Repeat in the opposite eye.
- Assess trigeminal branch sensation: after asking the patient to close the eyes, use a wisp of cotton wool to lightly touch the ophthalmic, maxillary and mandibular divisions on both sides of the face, and ask whether this can be felt.

Motor function (V)

- Ask the patient to clench the teeth, and feel the power of the masseter muscle just under the cheekbone on each side – the masseter muscle extends from the zygomatic arch in the cheek

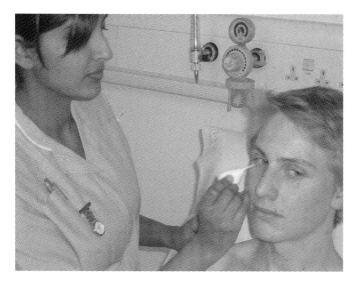

Fig 6.6 Eliciting the corneal reflex using tissue paper

to the mandible, is important in chewing and acts by closing the jaw (Marcovitch, 2005).

- Ask the patient to try and keep the mouth open whilst an attempt is made to close it – this tests the platysmus muscle. Look for discrepancies each side.
- Elicit the jaw jerk test (Figure 6.7).

Facial nerve (VII) motor function

- Note any facial paralysis, e.g. reduced wrinkling of the forehead, drooping at the corner of the mouth.
- Assess the power of the facial muscles by asking the patient to blow out the cheeks (whistle), to screw up the eyes, to frown, to raise the eyebrows and to grimace and show the teeth; using the fingers, check the muscle power for each manoeuvre and compare both sides.

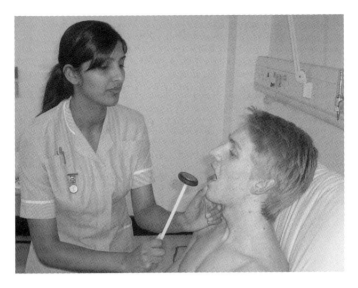

Fig 6.7 Eliciting the jaw jerk test

Examination of the vestibulocochlear nerve (VIII)

- Test the hearing of each ear (only the auditory part of the nerve is being tested).
- Place a hand over the patient's ear to avoid noise contamination.
- Rub the fingers of your other hand together next to the patient's other ear and ask whether this can be heard; alternatively, whisper a short sentence or a number and ask the patient to repeat it to you out loud.
- Repeat the above for the other ear.
- Ask the patient which side is loudest, or whether they are both the same.
- If hearing is impaired, use an auriscope to check each external ear passage and tympanic membrane (Figure 6.8).
- If there is any discrepancy between the ears, perform tuning fork tests.

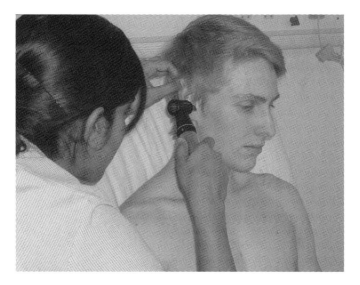

Fig 6.8 Using an auriscope to check the external ear passage and tympanic membrane

Rinne's test

In Rinne's test, air and bone conduction are tested using a 128 Hz tuning fork. Air conduction should be louder than bone conduction through the skull in a normal ear.

- Place a vibrating tuning fork next to the affected ear and ask the patient if it can be heard (Figure 6.9a).
- Then place the bottom end of a vibrating tuning fork on the mastoid process (Figure 6.9b) behind the ear and ask whether it is louder (bone conduction) than air conduction. If bone conduction is louder, this indicates a conductive deafness, which results from disease of the middle ear, e.g. otitis media. In neural deafness (i.e. disease of the VIIIth cranial nerve), both air and bone conduction will be quiet, but air conduction should still be louder than bone conduction.

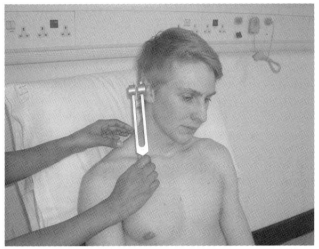

(a)

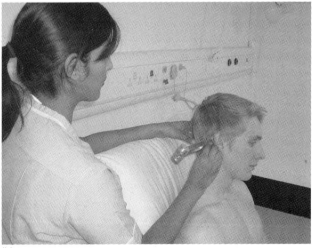

(b)

Fig 6.9 Rinne's test: place a vibrating tuning fork next to the affected ear and ask the patient if it can be heard (a); then place the bottom end of a vibrating tuning fork on the mastoid process (b) behind the ear and ask whether it is louder (bone conduction) than air conduction

Weber's test

- Place the base of a vibrating tuning fork on the middle of the forehead and ask the patient whether the sound is heard in the middle of the head or on one side of the head. In conductive deafness, the sound lateralizes towards the affected side (as a result of bone conduction), whereas, in neural deafness, the sound is heard louder on the unaffected side. This should confirm the findings from Rinne's test.

Examination of the glossopharyngeal and vagal nerves (IX, X)

- Ask the patient to say 'aahhh'.
- Using a pen-torch, observe the movements of the soft palate, uvula and posterior pharynx (Figure 6.10).

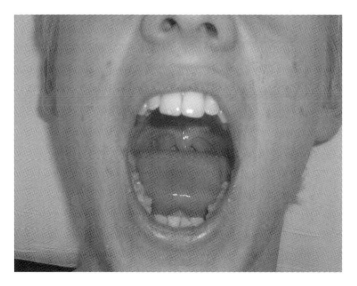

Fig 6.10 Observing the movements of the soft palate, uvula and posterior pharynx

Examination of the spinal accessory nerve (XI)

- Examine the trapezius and sternomastoid muscles in the neck.
- Ask the patient to shrug the shoulders against resistance (your hands).
- Push down on the shoulders to test the power in the trapezius muscle.
- Ask the patient to turn the head to the left; press against the left cheek and oppose the movement and feel the power in the opposite sternomastoid muscle. Repeat on the other side.

Examination of the hypoglossal nerve (XII)

- Ask the patient to open the mouth and note any wasting or fasciculation of lower motor neurone lesions on either side of the tongue.
- Ask the patient to stick out the tongue and note whether it deviates towards one side (indicating weakness on that side).
- Ask the patient to push the tongue into the left cheek and push against the cheek, whilst at the same time applying resistance using the fingers: assess the power and symmetry of movement (Ford *et al.*, 2005). Repeat on the other cheek.

EXAMINATION OF THE LOWER LIMBS

Diagnostic considerations

When performing a neurological examination of the lower limbs, the main diagnostic considerations are as follows:

- Does the patient have upper motor neurone or lower motor neurone signs, and are these signs bilateral (paraplegia) or unilateral (monoplegia)?
- Does the patient have a monoplegia with ipsilateral arm involvement (hemiplegia), accompanied by corresponding sensory loss (usually caused by a stroke or space-occupying lesion)?

Table 6.2 Comparison of motor weakness in upper and lower motor neurone lesions

Upper motor neurone lesions	Lower motor neurone lesions
Increased tone (spasticity)	Reduced tone (flaccidity)
Clonus (intermittent muscle relaxations and contractions)	
Reduced power in muscle groups	Reduced power in muscle groups
Hyperreflexia	Reflexes: diminished or absent
Extensor plantar response	Downwards plantar reflex
Muscle atrophy (wasting)	Pathological wasting (sometimes)
	Fasciculations

- Is there sensory loss without motor involvement.

The comparison of motor weakness in upper and lower motor neurone lesions is shown in Table 6.2.

Equipment
The following equipment is needed:

- Tendon hammer.
- Orange stick.
- Cotton wool.
- Neuro-tip.
- Tuning fork (128 Hz).

General considerations

- Ask the patient if there is pain anywhere in the body.
- Ask the patient to lie on an examination couch at 45°.
- Expose the patient below the waist, leaving on the underwear.

Assessment of gait

- If able, ask the patient to stand up; note whether the patient has ataxia (loss of coordination), the reasons for which include cerebellar disease causing loss of motor coordination (cerebellar ataxia) and loss of dorsal column joint position sense or proprioception in the feet (sensory ataxia).

- If the patient has ataxia, perform Romberg's test by asking the patient to stand with the feet together with the arms out in front and to close the eyes (stand close to the patient to prevent falling). If the patient becomes more unsteady on closing the eyes (positive for Romberg's test), sensory ataxia rather than cerebellar disease is present.

- Next, observe the patient's gait. Ask the patient to walk 10 paces towards you, to stop, turn around and walk back to the starting point. Look for the classic neurological gaits (Table 6.3) or any difficulties initiating movement or turning. If the patient is unsteady, stand close to prevent falling.

- Ask the patient to repeat the above, but walking heel-to-toe as if on a tight rope; this is not possible if the patient has ataxia (policeman asking intoxicated driver to walk in a straight line).

- Ask the patient to repeat the above, but walking on the heels; this is not possible if the patient has an L5 lesion and foot-drop.

- Ask the patient to repeat the above, but walking on 'tip-toes'; this is not possible if the patient has an S1 lesion.

Inspection of muscles

- Note the presence of muscle wasting; loss of muscle bulk is caused by long-term disuse atrophy of upper motor neurone lesions or wasting of lower motor neurone lesions.

- Note the presence of fasciculation (fine muscle twitching): occurs randomly at rest and stops during voluntary movements, suggesting lower motor neurone lesions (Ford *et al.*, 2005).

Assessment of tone

- Ask the patient to let the legs go 'floppy'. With the patient relaxed and the legs straight out on the bed, roll the leg medially and laterally to test tone.

Table 6.3 Classic neurological gaits

Cause	Characteristics
Parkinsonism	• Festinate (rapid, short and jerky steps as if falling forwards, chasing one's own centre of gravity • Shuffling, with difficulty initiating movement and turning • Bradykinesia (slow movement) and poor arm swing. Stooped posture with knees and hips bent
Steppage gait (high-stepping)	• The patient with a foot-drop cannot dorsiflex the foot; therefore, the knee has to be lifted up high to avoid toe scraping and the foot has to be 'slapped' down on the floor • Foot-drop is caused by common peroneal nerve palsy
Sensory ataxia (stamping)	• Lack of proprioception in both feet makes the patient unsteady (ataxic), and there is a reliance on visual attention to 'place' or 'stamp' each foot on the floor • The gait is wide based, ataxic with bilateral stamping and the patient is unable to walk heel-to-toe • Positive for Romberg's test – the gait can be normal with the eyes open
Cerebellar ataxia	• Jerky unsteadiness (ataxia) caused by loss of motor coordination from cerebellar disease • Wide based, ataxic with eyes open • Arms held out at sides to try and keep steady, often with a tremor • Unable to walk heel-to-toe and the patient falls to the side
Waddling gait (myopathic)	• Bilateral lower limb myopathy causes a characteristic waddling gait, like a duck • Pelvis drops when foot leaves the ground, toes touch the floor before the heels and the trunk moves side to side
Hemiplegic gait (foot-dragging)	• Unilateral spastic leg (old upper motor neurone lesion from a stroke) is held 'stiff' and slightly in extension • The patient is unable to bend the knee on walking, and subsequently scrapes the toe across the floor whilst describing a semicircle with the affected leg • Ipsilateral, spastic upper limb (held in flexion not extension)
Scissors gait	• Spastic paraparesis (bilateral upper motor neurone lesion) causes a scissors gait. Knees and hips are held slightly flexed in compensation • There is a stiff awkward scissoring motion as knees scrape each other • Also described as 'wading through mud'

- Jerk the leg upwards suddenly from under the knee: a leg with increased tone will not flex at the knee, but will fly up into the air.
- Check for patella clonus (clonus is sustained rhythmical contraction of a muscle after a sudden stretch, and is a sign of the hypertonia of upper motor neurone lesions): hold the patient's patella between the thumb and forefinger and pull down sharply; if patella clonus is present, this will elicit rhythmical contraction of the quadriceps.
- Check for ankle clonus: flex the knee slightly, and then perform a sustained but rapid dorsiflexion of the foot; if ankle clonus is present, this suggests an upper motor neurone lesion.

Assessment of power

- Test the power in the major muscle groups. Always ask the patients to do as much as possible themselves (this helps in the assessment of the muscle power against gravity in the leg and also against your own strength, thus allowing the power to be graded).
- Ask the patient to lift the leg off the bed without bending the knee (L2, L3 – hip flexors); test the power by pressing down on the thigh and asking the patient to resist the pressure (Figure 6.11).
- Test hip extension: place a hand under the patient's heel; ask the patient to straighten the leg and push the heel down on the hand (L4, L5 – hip extensors) (Figure 6.12).
- Test knee flexors: ask the patient to bend the knee and bring the heel up towards the bottom (L5, S1 – knee flexors); ask the patient to stop you from straightening the leg. Then, with the knee still bent, test knee extension: pull the heel out and try to straighten the leg. Ask the patient to push your hand away (L3, L4 – knee extensors).
- Test ankle plantar flexion: ask the patient to push against your hand – like pressing on a car accelerator (S1, S2 – ankle plantar flexion) (Figure 6.13a).

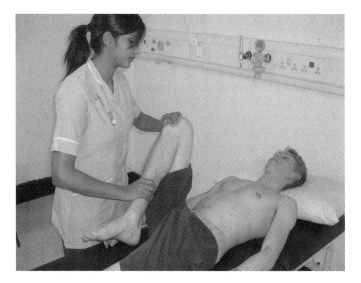

Fig 6.11 Assessing the power of hip flexion

- Test ankle dorsiflexion: ask the patient to cock the foot up against your hand (L4, L5 – ankle dorsiflexion) (Figure 6.13b).

Assessment of coordination

- Whilst running the hand down the right shin, ask the patient to put the left heel just below the right knee; repeat for the opposite side.
- Look for motor in-coordination; any abnormality may be caused by weakness of the legs, or may imply a cerebellar problem, i.e. cerebellar examination should be undertaken.

Assessment of spinal reflexes

A tendon hammer can be used to elicit spinal reflexes. If a reflex cannot be elicited, ask the patient to reinforce the reflex, e.g. ask the patient to clench the teeth when requested to do so. On prompting the patient, go ahead and try again. The following spinal reflexes should be assessed.

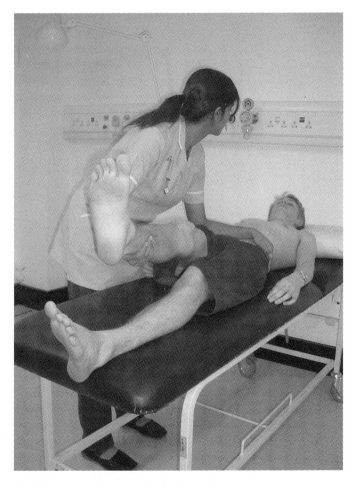

Fig 6.12 Assessing the power of hip extension

Knee jerk (L2, L3, L4 myotomes)

- Place one arm under the patient's knee and hold the hamstrings, with the knee slightly flexed.
- Ask the patient to relax.

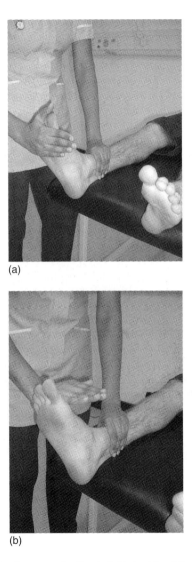

(a)

(b)

Fig 6.13 Assessing the power of ankle plantarflexion (a) and dorsiflexion (b)

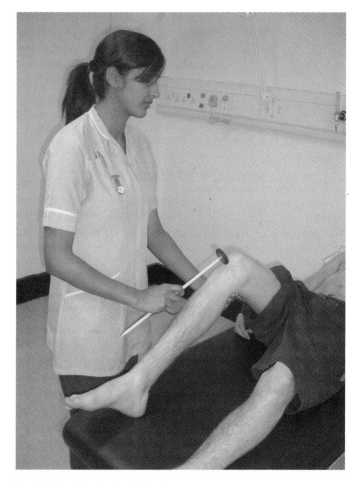

Fig 6.14 Assessing the knee jerk reflex

- With the tendon hammer in the dominant hand, tap the ligament below the patella (rather than the patella itself) two or three times (Figure 6.14). Reflexes can be classified as normal, brisk (hyperreflexia), diminished (hyporeflexia) or absent.

Ankle jerk (S1, S2)

- Dorsiflex the ankle with the knee slightly flexed and the hip externally rotated.

Babinski reflex (plantar reflex)

- Using the orange stick, drag the point of the stick from the heel up the outer part of the sole and around under the great toe. The normal response is a down-going plantar reflex. A positive Babinski reflex, otherwise known as an extensor plantar response, may be observed if there is an upper motor neurone lesion.

Assessment of sensation

The different modalities of sensation need to be examined because not all are affected at the same time. Light touch, vibration and proprioception are dorsal column functions, whereas pain and temperature are spinothalamic functions. Each dermatome from L2 to S2 needs to be tested (Figure 6.15), and it is important to remember that peripheral nerve lesions commonly present in a 'glove (arms) and stocking (legs)' distribution, e.g. diabetic neuropathy. This results in a sensory level on each leg that does not necessarily conform to dermatomes, and may not be the same on both sides.

Light touch

- Demonstrate the light touch sensation test to the patient: using cotton wool, dab lightly on the sternum and ask whether this can be felt.
- Perform the test on each dermatome from L2 to S2 (Figure 6.15).
- Ask the patient whether it feels the same as the test on the chest or whether it is different; note any areas where it differs.

Vibration

- Perform the vibration sense test using a 128 Hz tuning fork.

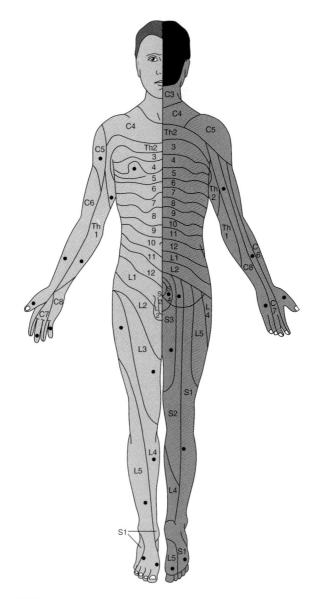

Fig 6.15 Dermatomes

- Demonstrate the vibration sensation test to the patient: strike the tuning fork on your forearm or hand (not the patient's) and place the round end on the sternum, checking that the patient can feel the vibration; if the vibration is felt, proceed with the test.
- Reactivate the tuning fork and place on the end of the great toe (Figure 6.16): if the patient can feel it vibrating (rather than just light touch), ask when the sensation stops (actively stop the tuning fork from vibrating and check whether the patient notices).
- If the patient cannot feel the vibration on the great toe, repeat the test on a more proximal bony landmark: the first metatarsophalangeal joint first, then the ankle joint if necessary and, finally, the patella of the knee.
- Document the position at which the patient first senses the vibration.

Proprioception

- Test joint position sense (proprioception) on the interphalangeal joint of the great toe.
- Ask the patient to close the eyes.
- Isolate the distal great toe joint by positioning the thumb and index finger of the left hand either side of the toe at a point just proximal to the joint and the thumb and index finger of the right hand either side distal to the joint. Take care not to hold the dorsum or plantar aspect of the toes, because this could indicate to the patient where the pressure is being applied.
- Bend the distal toe upwards and then downwards; advise the patient what is being done and ask whether it can be felt (if the answer is yes, perform further random up and down movements of the toe and ask the patient to confirm when and which way the great toe is being moved; this will help to ensure the accuracy of the test).
- If the patient's joint position sense in the great toe is impaired, isolate a more proximal joint (ankle; then, if necessary, the knee).

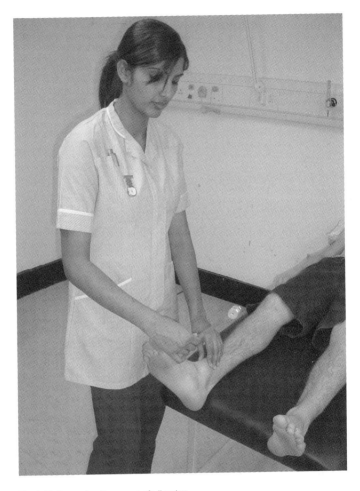

Fig 6.16 Assessing the sense of vibration

Pain

- Using a neuro-tip, demonstrate the pain sensation test on the patient's sternum.
- When testing each dermatome, ask the patient whether the pin feels sharp, the pain sensation changes or the pain ceases altogether.

EXAMINATION OF THE UPPER LIMBS

Diagnostic considerations

When undertaking a neurological examination of the upper limbs, the main diagnostic considerations are as follows:

- Does the patient have upper motor neurone or lower motor neurone signs?
- Are these signs bilateral (paraplegia) or unilateral (monoplegia)?
- Is there sensory loss without motor involvement.
- Does the patient have a radial, ulnar or median nerve palsy (these are also peripheral nerve lesions).

Equipment

- Tendon hammer.
- Cotton wool.
- A piece of paper.
- Neuro-tip.
- Tuning fork (128 Hz).

Inspection of muscles

- Observe the upper limbs for loss of muscle bulk (results from long-term disuse atrophy of upper motor neurone lesions or wasting of lower motor neurone lesions); note which parts of the hand are wasted: thenar and/or hypothenar wasting.
- Observe for fasciculation (fine twitching of muscle groups in lower motor neurone lesions).

- Test for pronator drift (a subtle sign of upper motor neurone weakness): a difference in the muscular tone between pronation (bones of the forearm are crossed and the palm of the hand faces downwards) and supination (turning of the forearm and hand so that the palm faces upwards) causes the affected arm to pronate when the eyes are closed; ask the patient to close the eyes and put the arms straight out in front with the palms upwards. Look for pronation of the arm with the eyes closed.
- Look for the resting tremor of parkinsonism; postural and intention tremors will be evident during examination of coordination.

Assessment of tone

- Ask the patient to relax and let the arms go 'floppy'.
- Passively flex and extend the wrist repeatedly; then make a circular motion with the hand specifically to look for cogwheeling (rigidity plus resting tremor) of parkinsonism.
- Repeat the above at the elbow and shoulder by flexing and extending.

Assessment of power

- Test the power of the shoulders.
- Sit the patient forward with the arms out to the sides, the shoulders abducted at 90° to the body and the elbows fully flexed (a demonstration of this may be required).
- Apply downwards pressure over the elbow of one outstretched arm; ask the patient to resist this (testing C5 – shoulder abduction) (abduction = move away from the mid-line).
- Apply upwards pressure from beneath the elbow of one outstretched arm; ask the patient to resist this (testing C6 – shoulder adduction) (adduction = move towards the mid-line).
- Repeat the above for the other outstretched arm.
- Test the power of the elbows.
- Ask the patient to position the arms straight out in front, with the elbows flexed; ask the patient to clench the fists – 'boxing guard'.

- Try to straighten out the arm; ask the patient to resist this (testing C5, C6 – elbow flexion).
- Then ask the patient to try to straighten the arm whilst you attempt to prevent this (testing C7, C8 – elbow extension).
- Test the power of the wrist and hand. Here, the myotomes overlap with peripheral nerve function of the median, ulnar and radial nerves, which share the same nerve roots. Therefore, median, ulnar and radial nerve functions are being screened.
- Ask the patient to make a fist and cock the wrist back; try to bend the wrist down; ask the patient to resist this (testing C6, C7 and radial nerve – wrist extension).
- Ask the patient to straighten the fingers; try to bend the fingers down; ask the patient to resist this (testing C7, C8 and radial nerve – finger extension).
- Offer the patient two fingers to squeeze (testing C7, C8 – finger flexion); this also allows an assessment of overall hand function and whether the patient can undertake activities of daily living.
- Ask the patient to spread the fingers apart; try to push them together; ask the patient to resist this (testing T1 – ulnar nerve).
- Ask the patient to hold a piece of paper between the fingers; try to pull the paper out of the fingers; ask the patient to resist this (testing T1 – ulnar nerve).
- Perform a specific median nerve test; ask the patient to oppose the thumb and little finger. Try to pull them apart; ask the patient to resist this (testing median nerve opposes the thumb – opponens policis).

Assessment of coordination
Finger–nose test
Hold up a finger in front of the patient and keep it still.

- Ask the patient to repeatedly touch the nose and then your finger (not too quickly): observe for tremor and in-coordination.

Assessment of spinal reflexes

A tendon hammer can be used to elicit spinal reflexes. If a reflex cannot be elicited, ask the patient to reinforce the reflex, e.g. ask the patient to clench the teeth when requested to do so. On prompting the patient, go ahead and try again. The following spinal reflexes should be assessed.

Biceps jerk (C5, C6)

- Rest the patient's arm across the lower part of the chest so that the elbow is flexed at roughly 90°; ensure that the muscles are relaxed.
- Position the thumb over the biceps tendon and strike it with the tendon hammer (striking the thumb helps to augment the response and avoids causing pain to the patient) (Figure 6.17).
- Observe for contraction of the biceps or flexion of the elbow.

Triceps jerk (C7, C8)

- Maintain the position described above, but with the thumb positioned on the triceps tendon.
- Strike the thumb with the tendon hammer.
- Observe for extension of the elbow or contraction of the triceps.
- Some practitioners prefer to strike the tendon directly (Figure 6.18).

Supinator (C5, C6, C7)

- Maintain the position described above.
- Locate the brachioradialis tendon at the wrist; if unable to locate it, place two fingers perpendicular to the wrist, at a point just proximal to the watchstrap: this correlates with the location of the tendon.
- Strike the fingers with the tendon hammer.
- Observe for adduction at the wrist or contraction of the brachioradialis.

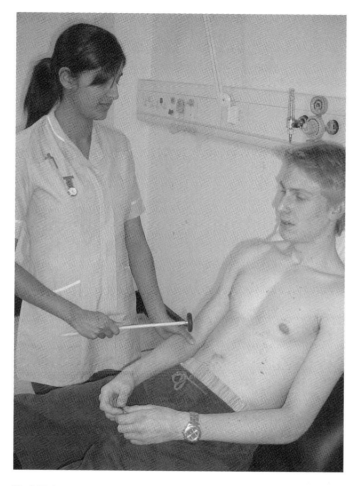

Fig 6.17 Assessing the biceps jerk

Assessment of sensation

The different modalities of sensation need to be examined because not all are affected at the same time. Light touch, vibration and proprioception are dorsal column functions, whereas pain and

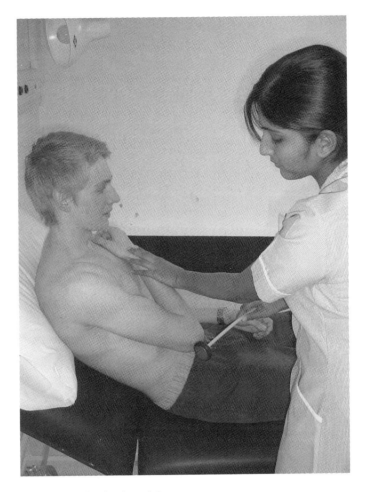

Fig 6.18 Assessing the triceps jerk

temperature are spinothalamic functions. Each dermatome from C5 to T2 needs to be tested (Figure 6.15).

Light touch

- Demonstrate the light touch sensation test to the patient: using cotton wool, dab lightly on the sternum and ask whether this can be felt.
- Perform the test on each dermatome from C5 to T2 (Figure 6.15).
- Ask the patient whether it feels the same as the test on the chest or whether it is different; note any areas where it differs.

Vibration

- Perform the vibration sense test using a 128 Hz tuning fork.
- Demonstrate the vibration sensation test to the patient: strike the tuning fork on your forearm or hand (not the patient's) and place the round end on the sternum, checking that the patient can feel the vibration; if the vibration is felt, proceed with the test.
- Reactivate the tuning fork and place on the end of the index finger: if the patient can feel it vibrating (rather than just light touch), ask when the sensation stops (actively stop the tuning fork from vibrating and check whether the patient notices).
- If the patient cannot feel the vibration on the index finger, repeat the test on a more proximal bony landmark: index finger metacarpophalangeal joint first, then the wrist joint if necessary and, finally, the elbow.
- Document the position at which the patient first senses the vibration.

Proprioception

- Test joint position sense (proprioception) on the index finger.
- Ask the patient to close the eyes.
- Isolate the distal interphalangeal joint of the index finger by positioning the thumb and index finger of the left hand either

side of the finger at a point just proximal to the joint and the thumb and index finger of the right hand either side distal to the joint. Take care not to hold the dorsum or plantar aspect of the finger, because this could indicate to the patient where pressure is being applied.

- Bend the distal phalanx upwards and then downwards; advise the patient what is being done and ask whether it can be felt (if the answer is yes, perform further random up and down movements of the finger and ask the patient to confirm when and which way the finger is being moved; this will help to ensure the accuracy of the test).

- If the patient's joint position sense in the finger is impaired, isolate a more proximal joint (wrist; then, if necessary, the elbow).

Pain

- Using a neuro-tip, demonstrate the pain sensation test on the patient's sternum.

- When testing each dermatome, ask the patient whether the pin feels sharp, the pain sensation changes or the pain ceases altogether.

EXAMINATION OF THE CEREBELLUM

Examination of the cerebellum is an examination routine in its own right. Some aspects of the examination, e.g. coordination, are usually undertaken during examination of the lower and upper limbs. This is a more detailed examination to look for motor incoordination. It is important to remember that the signs are continuous with the affected (ipsilateral) side of the cerebellum, and so both sides should be compared at all times: bilateral disease causes bilateral signs. It may be helpful to remember the mnemonic 'DANISH PR':

- **D**ysdiadochokinesia: clumsy, disorganized rapid alternating movements; loss of the ability to perform rapid alternate movements, e.g. winding up a watch (Marcovitch, 2005).
- **A**taxic gait (wide based).

- **N**ystagmus towards the side of the lesion.
- **I**ntention tremor on finger–nose testing, but not at rest!
- **S**lurred speech: 'staccato' or 'scanning' dysarthria, i.e. halting and jerky.
- **H**ypotonia (generalized reduced muscle tone).
- **P**ast pointing on finger–nose testing: pointing past the finger.
- **R**ebound overshooting with eyes closed.

It is not practical to examine the cerebellum in this order, and so the following routine is suggested:

- Ask the patient whether there is any pain.
- Expose the patient to the waist.
- Ask the patient to stand up and examine the gait, looking for ataxia (described in section on 'Examination of the lower limbs', pp. 139–140).
- Ask the patient to sit back down.
- Ask the patient to tap the back of the right hand into the palm of the left hand repeatedly (this desensitizes the cerebellum); then ask the patient to turn the right hand over and back repeatedly to test for dysdiadochokinesia.
- Ask the patient to hold the arms out in front and close the eyes; then tap one hand downwards slightly and look for overshooting on recoil.
- Examine the muscle tone in each upper limb.
- Use finger–nose testing for intention tremor and past pointing (see p. 153).
- Observe for horizontal nystagmus only (not vertical).
- Observe for scanning dysarthria only (not dysphasia).

Assessment of higher mental function

The assessment of higher mental function is important to recognize patients with acute delirium (acute confusional state) or cognitive decline of dementia. Hodgkinson's Abbreviated Mental Test Score (AMTS) (Hodgkinson, 1972) is used widely to rapidly assess patients for whom there is a clinical suspicion of dementia. It is also now used to establish a diagnosis of acute confusion on admission to hospital and to monitor response to treatment.

Box 6.2 The Abbreviated Mental Test Score (AMTS)

Question	Score
What is your age?	0 or 1
What is the time (to the nearest hour)?	0 or 1
Give the patient an address, e.g. '42 West Street', and ask him/her to repeat it at the end of the test. Ask the patient to repeat the address to ensure that it has been heard correctly	
What is the year?	0 or 1
What is the name of the hospital or number of the residence in which you are situated?	0 or 1
Can you recognize two persons (the doctor, nurse, home help, etc.)?	0 or 1
What is your date of birth?	0 or 1
In which year did the First World War begin (adjust this for a world event that the patient would have known during childhood)?	0 or 1
What is the name of the present monarch (head of state, etc.)?	0 or 1
Count backwards from 20 to 1	0 or 1
Repeat address	0 or 1
Score/10	

(After Hodgkinson, 1972)

(Reproduced with permission from Oxford University Press from Hodkinson, 1972)

The AMTS takes 1 min to carry out and involves asking the patient a set of questions (Box 6.2). Each correctly answered question scores one point; a score of less than 7 suggests abnormal cognitive function (Jitapunkul *et al.*, 1991). In dementia, more formal tests are necessary to confirm the diagnosis.

Examination of speech

There are a number of routine questions that can be used to distinguish between the neurological disorders of speech: dysphasia and dysarthria. Dysphasia is the term used to describe difficulties in understanding language and in self-expression, usually seen

Table 6.4 Classification of dysphasia

Type	Characteristics	Area
Receptive dysphasia	Fluent, unintelligible jargon No insight No comprehension	Wernicke's area Dominant frontal lobe
Expressive dysphasia	Normal comprehension Insight – frustrated Word-finding difficulties Lacks fluency	Broca's area Dominant parietal lobe
Global aphasia	Receptive and expressive dysphasia	Suggests whole dominant middle cerebral artery territory

---

Box 6.3 Causes of dysarthria

- Non-specific causes, e.g. hypothyroidism, confusion.
- Bulbar speech (nasal, slurred consonants) from bulbar cranial *lower* motor neurones.
- Pseudobulbar speech (high-pitched 'Donald Duck') from bulbar cranial *upper* motor neurones.
- Cerebellar (staccato, scanning).
- Deafness (nasal).
- Orofacial dyspraxia: difficulties in making the phonic shapes needed for speech. In autism and frontal lobe dementia.

---

following a stroke or other cerebral damage (Marcovitch, 2005). The classification of dysphasia is given in Table 6.4. Dysarthria is the term used when weakness or in-coordination of the speech musculature prevents the clear pronunciation of words; the patient's speech may sound slurred or weak ((Marcovitch, 2005). The causes of dysarthria are listed in Box 6.3.

Testing for dysphasia

- Encourage patients to talk. Ask them to say their name, where they live, what they had for breakfast, the names of their grandchildren, etc.

- Try to recognize receptive or expressive dysphasia: if comprehension is impaired, there is receptive dysphasia, but, if comprehension is good, there is no receptive element.
- To test comprehension, perform a few simple commands (without gesturing), e.g. 'please put out your tongue', 'please shut your eyes' or 'please touch your nose'. Proceed to look for expressive dysphasia: ask the patient to name a few objects, e.g. a pen, a watch or a cup, and look for word-finding difficulties.

Testing for dysarthria

- Examine more closely for dysarthria by asking the patient to repeat a few difficult phrases: 'baby hippopotamus', 'West Register Street' and 'British Constitution'.

CONCLUSION

In this chapter, the examination of the neurological system has been described. A methodical approach, incorporating an assessment of the conscious level, examination of the cranial nerves, examination of the limbs and examination of the cerebellum, has been discussed.

REFERENCES

Cox N, Roper T (2005) *Clinical Skills: Oxford Core Text*. Oxford University Press, Oxford.

Ford M, Hennessey I, Japp A (2005) *Introduction to Clinical Examination*. Elsevier, Oxford.

Gleadle J (2004) *History and Examination at a Glance*. Blackwell Publishing, Oxford.

Hodgkinson H (1972) Evaluation of a mental test score for assessment of mental impairment in the elderly. *Age Ageing* **1**: 233–238.

Jennet B, Teasdale, G (1974) Assessment of coma and impaired consciousness. A practical scale. *Lancet* **ii**: 81–83.

Jitapunkul S, Pillay I, Ebrahim S (1991) The abbreviated mental test: its use and validity. *Age Ageing* **20**: 332–336.

Mackay C, Burke D, Burke J, Porter K, Bowden D, Gorman D (2000) Association between the assessment of conscious level using the AVPU system and the Glasgow coma scale. *Pre-hospital Immediate Care* **4**: 17–19.

Marcovitch H (2005) *Black's Medical Dictionary*, 41st edn. A & C Black, London.

National Institute for Clinical Excellence (NICE) (2007) *Head Injury: Triage, Assessment, Investigation and Early Management of Head Injuries in Infants, Children and Adults, Clinical Guideline No. 56*. NICE, London. Available at www.nice.org.uk [accessed on 16 April 2008].

Resuscitation Council UK (2006) *Immediate Life Support Manual*, 2nd edn. Resuscitation Council UK, London.

Examination of the Musculoskeletal System

7

Yi-Yang Ng

INTRODUCTION

Musculoskeletal or rheumatological problems are common and can cause significant morbidity. Diagnosis can be made following detailed history taking, sound physical examination and, where indicated, appropriate investigations, e.g. X-rays.

The examination of the musculoskeletal system involves the look (inspection), feel (palpation) and move (active and passive) approach. In addition, special tests can be performed on certain joints to elicit further clinical features to aid in the diagnosis. Neurological assessment of the upper and lower limbs forms part of the spinal examination, and is described in Chapter 6.

The chapter's author would like to stress that the examination techniques for the knee, hip and shoulder joints are described in detail, but those for the hand, wrist, back, ankle and foot are only outlined briefly; if a more detailed account is required, reference to an authoritative orthopaedic textbook is suggested.

The aim of this chapter is to provide an understanding of the principles of examination of the musculoskeletal system.

LEARNING OUTCOMES

At the end of this chapter, the reader will be able to:

❏ List the symptoms of musculoskeletal disease.
❏ Discuss the examination of the knee joint.
❏ Discuss the examination of the hip joint.
❏ Discuss the examination of the shoulder joint.
❏ Briefly outline the examination of the ankle and foot.
❏ Briefly outline the examination of the wrist and hand.
❏ Briefly outline the examination of the spine.

SYMPTOMS OF MUSCULOSKELETAL DISEASE

The symptoms of musculoskeletal disease include:

- Weakness.
- Joint stiffness.
- Joint pain.
- Joint swelling.
- Hot joints.
- Mobility problems.
- Loss of function.

(Sources: Gleadle, 2004; Ford *et al.*, 2005)

EXAMINATION OF THE KNEE JOINT

Relevant anatomy

The knee joint is made up of four bones:

- Patella.
- Femur.
- Tibia.
- Fibula.

There are four ligaments (anterior cruciate ligament, posterior cruciate ligament, medial collateral ligament and lateral collateral ligament) present in the knee joint, which provide strength and stability to the joint. The menisci (cartilages situated within the knee joint) serve to protect the ends of the bones from rubbing against each other and act as shock absorbers (Moore & Dalley, 2006). The main movements of the knee joint are flexion and extension.

Injury to the knee joint

The 'unhappy triad' commonly occurs in contact sports, such as football, when the knee is hit from the outside. This results in injury to the anterior cruciate ligament, medial collateral ligament and medial meniscus (Moore & Dalley, 2006).

Procedure for examination of the knee joint

The examination of the knee joint should be undertaken thoroughly and systematically following the 'look, feel and move' approach.

Look

With patient standing:

- Expose the patient's knees and thighs.
- Look at the knees from the front, sides and behind: check for genu varum (bow-legs), genu valgum (knock-knees), genu recurvatum (knee hyperextension) and abnormality at the popliteal fossa.
- Assess the patient's gait. A single sequence of functions of one limb is called a gait cycle. The gait cycle has two basic units: the stance phase (when the limb is in contact with the ground) and the swing phase (when the foot is in the air for limb advancement). An antalgic gait refers to a characteristic gait resulting from pain on weight-bearing, in which the stance phase of gait is shortened on the affected side (Douglas *et al.*, 2005).

With patient lying supine:

- Compare both knees and look for gross deformity, skin changes, scars and swelling.
- If wasting of the quadriceps is suspected, measure the circumference of the muscle 15 cm proximal to the tibial tuberosity; compare the measurement with the opposite side (Douglas *et al.*, 2005).
- Squat down and inspect from the side of each knee to assess fixed flexion deformity, suggested by a gap between the knee and the bed, i.e. the patient cannot extend the affected knee.

Feel

- Check whether the knee joint is painful prior to palpation; if it is, examine the other one first.

- Run the back of the hand along the joint to check the skin temperature (a warm skin temperature suggests possible infection or inflammation).
- Ask the patient to bend the knee at approximately 30°.
- Feel the patient's medial and lateral joint lines and palpate along the collateral ligaments for tenderness (Figure 7.1).
- Feel the patella and patella ligament.
- Feel the popliteal fossa for abnormal swelling, e.g. Baker's cyst, and popliteal aneurysm.

Move

- Evaluate active movements of both knee joints: ask the patient to bend the knee (flexion) and extend the knee (extension); the normal range of movement of both knee joints is between 0° (extension) and 140° (flexion) (Ford *et al.*, 2005).
- Evaluate passive movements of both knee joints: rest one hand on the patient's knee cap and flex and extend the knee with the other. Note the range of movement and whether crepitus is present.

Testing for knee effusion

- *Bulge test* (useful for the detection of mild to moderate effusion) (Douglas *et al.*, 2005): use one hand to massage any fluid away from the medial side of the knee. Then, use the other hand to massage along the lateral side of the knee and check whether there is a bulge occurring on the medial side.
- *Patellar tap test* (useful for the detection of gross effusion) (Douglas *et al.*, 2005): use one hand to massage any fluid away from the medial side of the knee. Then, use the other hand to apply firm pressure, starting from the proximal thigh to just above the knee cap. Whilst maintaining firm pressure, use the other hand's index and middle fingers to press the patella. If fluid is present, the patella will bounce off.

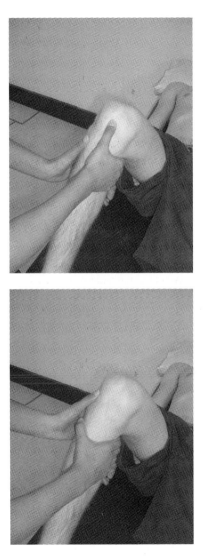

Fig 7.1 Palpation of the knee: feel the patient's medial and lateral joint lines and palpate along the collateral ligaments for tenderness

Evaluating the integrity of the collateral ligaments

- Flex the knee at approximately 30°.
- Evaluate the medial collateral ligament: support the lateral aspect of the knee with one hand and push medially with the other hand on the lower leg near the ankle (Figure 7.2a). Movement of more than 5–10° indicates laxity (Cox & Roper, 2005).
- Evaluate the lateral collateral ligament: support the medial aspect of the knee with one hand and push medially with the other hand on the lower leg near the ankle (Figure 7.2b). Movement of more than 5–10° indicates laxity (Cox & Roper, 2005).
- Repeat the above for the opposite knee.

Evaluating the integrity of the cruciate ligaments

- Flex the knee at 90° and sit very close to the patient's foot.
- Evaluate the anterior cruciate ligament: position both thumbs on the joint lines with the fingers wrapped around the tibia and pull the tibia away from the patient (Figure 7.3a); movement of more than 5–10° indicates laxity (Cox & Roper, 2005).
- Evaluate the posterior cruciate ligament: position both thumbs on the joint lines with the fingers wrapped around the tibia and push the tibia towards the patient (Figure 7.3b); movement of more than 5–10° indicates laxity (Cox & Roper, 2005).
- Repeat the above for the opposite knee.

Testing the integrity of the menisci

> NB: this test may cause significant discomfort to the patient if there is underlying meniscal disease.

- Position the patient in a prone position.
- Flex the knee at 90°.
- Stabilize the patient's hamstring with one hand at the popliteal fossa and hold the patient's foot with the other.

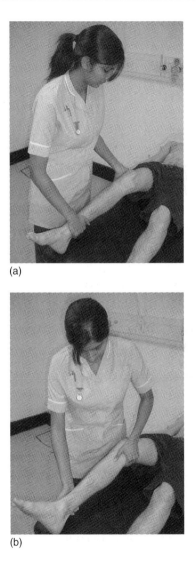

(a)

(b)

Fig 7.2 Assessing the medial collateral ligament (a) and lateral collateral ligament (b)

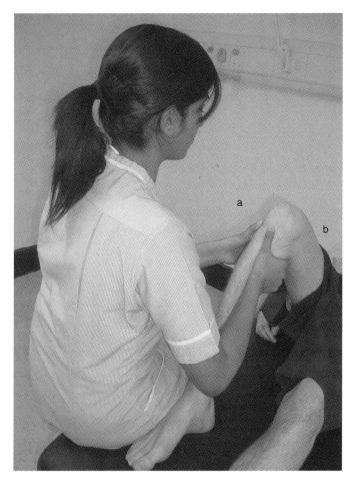

Fig 7.3 Assessing the anterior cruciate ligament (a) and posterior cruciate ligament (b)

- Twist the foot in a grinding motion. A grinding sensation and/or pain indicates meniscal damage (Kesson & Atkins, 2005).
- Repeat the above for the opposite knee.

All knee examinations should be accompanied by a hip examination as they share the same nerve supply.

EXAMINATION OF THE HIP JOINT

Anatomy
The hip joint is a ball and socket synovial joint formed by the articulation of the rounded head of the femur and the cup-like acetabulum of the pelvis. The surface of the femoral head and the inside of the acetabulum are covered with articular cartilage. Articular cartilage is a tough, slick material that allows the surfaces to slide against one another without damage. The hip joint is a weight-bearing joint which forms the primary connection between the bones of the lower limb and the axial skeleton of the trunk and pelvis.

Osteoarthritis of the hip joints
Osteoarthritis, also known as wear-and-tear arthritis or degenerative joint disease, is characterized by progressive 'wearing away' of the protective articular cartilage of the joint by hip arthritis, exposing bare bone within the joint. This condition typically affects patients aged over 50 years, especially those who are overweight and those who have suffered previous trauma to the hip and fractures to the bone around the joint. There is also a familial tendency to this condition. Classical symptoms of degenerative hip arthritis include pain on walking, stiffness, reduced range of motion and limp.

Procedure for examination of the hip joint
Look
With patient standing:

- Expose the patient's lower limbs.
- Look from the front, sides and behind the hips.

- Note any swelling, deformity, scars and gluteal wasting.
- Assess the patient's gait.

With patient lying supine:

- Using a tape measure, assess the apparent leg length from the xiphisternum (or umbilicus) to the medial malleolus and the true leg length from the anterior superior iliac spine to the medial malleolus. A difference in apparent leg length is caused by pelvic tilting and hip pathology on the shorter side in true leg length.

Feel

- Palpate both sides at the groin creases for tenderness.
- Palpate over the greater trochanters; then position the thumbs over the anterior superior iliac spines and the index/middle fingers over the tips of the greater trochanters. If one side is higher than the other, the higher side is abnormal.

Move

With the patient lying supine:

- Evaluate active movements of the hip joint.
- Ask the patient to bring the knee towards the chest (flexion).
- Ask the patient to move a straight leg away from the mid-line (abduction) (Figure 7.4).
- Ask the patient to move a straight leg across the mid-line (adduction) (Figure 7.5).
- Ask the patient to turn the foot outwards (external rotation).
- Ask the patient to turn the foot inwards (internal rotation).
- Repeat the above for the other hip joint.

With the patient lying prone:

- Evaluate passive movements of the hip joint.
- Evaluate flexion of the hip: push the knee towards the patient's body (flexion); the range of movement should be less than 120°.

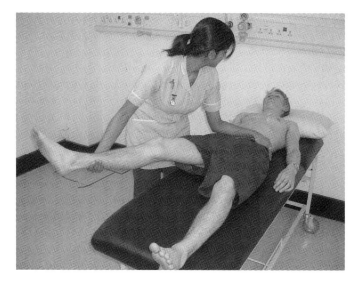

Fig 7.4 Assessing hip abduction

- Evaluate abduction of the hip: stabilize the pelvis by placing one arm across the anterior superior iliac spines and support the patient's calf muscle with the hand of the other arm and draw the leg away from the mid-line; once the pelvis starts to move forwards, it indicates maximal hip abduction; the range of movement should be less than 45°.
- Evaluate adduction of the hip: with the pelvis stabilized, move the patient's leg away across the mid-line; the range of movement should be less than 30°.
- Evaluate internal and external rotation of the hip: flex the hip and knee joints at 90°. Internal rotation: rotate the foot laterally, thereby turning the hip inwards (Figure 7.6). External rotation: rotate the foot medially, thereby turning the hip outwards (Figure 7.7). The range of movement should be less than 45° in both directions.

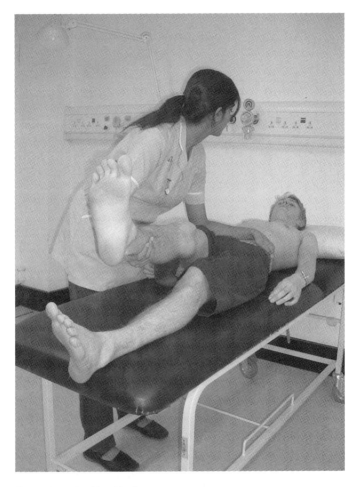

Fig 7.5 Assessing hip adduction

- Evaluate extension of the hip: lift the thigh up off the bed by pulling the foot upwards; the range of movement should be up to 30°.
- Repeat the above for the other hip joint.

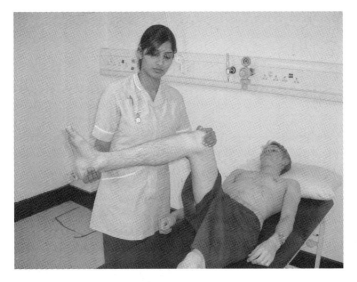

Fig 7.6 Assessing internal rotation of the hip

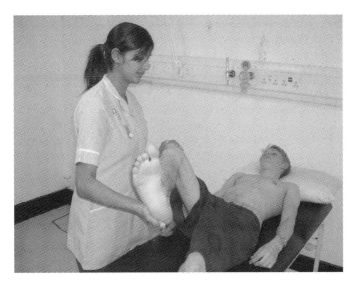

Fig 7.7 Assessing external rotation of the hip

177

Special tests

Thomas' hip flexion test

Thomas' hip flexion test is used to illustrate fixed flexion deformity of the hip (Talley & O'Connor, 2006).

- With the patient lying supine, place one hand beneath the patient's lumbar spine to ensure that it remains flat during the procedure.
- Using the other hand, flex the patient's hip and observe the opposite hip; in the presence of fixed flexion deformity, the opposite hip will flex following this manoeuvre.
- Repeat the above for the other hip.

Trendelenburg test

The Trendelenburg test is used to check the abductor function of the hip.

- Whilst in a standing position, ask the patient to place the hands on yours for support.
- Ask the patient to stand on one leg and observe the pelvis, noting the direction of tilt (Figure 7.8); normally, the pelvis will rise on the side of the leg which is lifted. In the presence of hip pathology with instability, the pelvis may drop on the side of the leg which is lifted.
- Repeat the above for the other hip.

EXAMINATION OF THE SHOULDER JOINT

Anatomy

The shoulder joint, a ball and socket synovial joint, is formed between the hemispherical head of the humerus and the shallow glenoid fossa. The joint capsule is strengthened by the surrounding ligaments and the rotator cuff muscles (subscapularis, supraspinatus, infraspinatus and teres minor) which provide stability. The lack of muscle inferiorly accounts for frequent downward dislocation (Abrahams *et al.*, 2005).

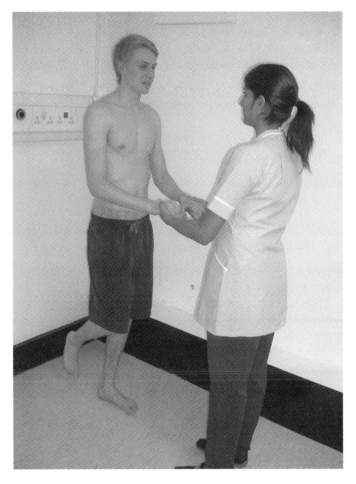

Fig 7.8 The Trendelenburg test: used to check the abductor function of the hip

Conditions affecting the shoulder joint

Anterior dislocation of the shoulder is a common injury, usually resulting from a blow on the fully abducted arm. Frequent dislocation may be the result of damage to the shoulder capsule and rotator cuff muscles. Degenerative tendonitis of the rotator cuff is common and affects elderly people in particular. This may result in a painful arc of shoulder abduction, occasionally restricting all movement. The serratus anterior muscle is paralysed as a result of long thoracic nerve injury. When pushing with the palms against a wall, the affected medial border of the scapula moves laterally and posteriorly away from the thoracic wall, giving the scapula the appearance of a wing (Moore & Dalley, 2006).

Procedure for examination of the shoulder joint

- Ask the patient to remove the clothes from the top half of the body in order to expose the shoulders.

Look

- Compare both sides.
- Look for muscle wasting (especially deltoid), scars, swelling, deformity and asymmetry.

Feel

- Palpate all over the shoulder (sternoclavicular joint, clavicle, acromioclavicular joint, acromial process, head of humerus, coracoid process, spine of scapula and greater tuberosity of humerus) for swelling and tenderness, and assess the muscle bulk of the deltoid.

Move

- Evaluate active movements of the shoulder.
- Ask the patient to move the arm upwards (flexion); the normal range of movement is 180°.
- Ask the patient to move the arm backwards as far as possible (extension); the normal range of movement is 65°.
- Ask the patient to move the arm laterally away from the body until the fingers point to the ceiling (abduction); the normal range of movement is 180°.

- From abduction, ask the patient to swing the arm across the trunk (adduction); the normal range of movement is 50°.
- Ask the patient to bend the elbow at 90° and move the hands as far apart as possible (external rotation); the normal range of movement is 65°.
- Ask the patient to bend the elbow at 90° and move the hands as close to each other as possible (internal rotation); the normal range of movement is 90°.
- Evaluate passive movements of the shoulder.
- Repeat all the range of movements described above by moving the arm for the patient.
- Check for limitation and/or discomfort and whether crepitus is present.
- Repeat the above for the other shoulder.

Special tests

Test for a painful arc

- With the patient's shoulder in full abduction, passively adduct the shoulder through an arc of 180°; in a rotator cuff injury, classically, the transition from 120° to 40° is painful (Douglas *et al.*, 2005).
- Repeat the above for the other shoulder.

Test for supraspinatus tendonitis

- Ask the patient to abduct the shoulder against resistance using the force of the hand (Figure 7.9); the movement will be painful in the presence of supraspinatus tendonitis.
- Repeat the above for the other shoulder.

EXAMINATION OF THE ANKLE AND FOOT

- Ask the patient to take off the shoes and socks in order to expose the feet and ankles. Compare both sides.

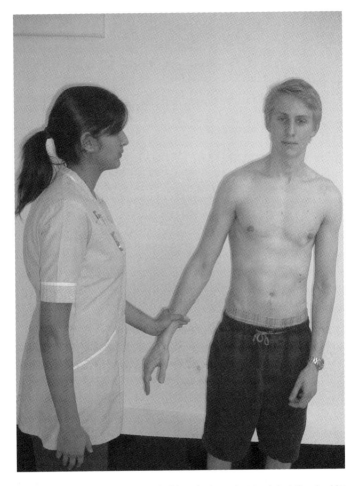

Fig 7.9 Test for supraspinatus tendonitis: ask the patient to abduct the shoulder against resistance using the force of the hand

Look

With the patient standing:

- Look for scars, deformity, swelling, pes cavus (high arched foot) and pes plantus (flat foot).

With the patient lying supine:

- Look for ulcers and callus (especially on the sole of the foot).
- Inspect the toes for abnormality of the toenails, hallux valgus (fixed lateral deviation of the main axis of the great toe), clawing (fixed flexion deformity of the toe) and crowding of the toes.

Feel

- Feel for swelling around the ankle, especially over the medial and lateral malleoli (Douglas *et al.*, 2005).
- Using the thumb and fingers, squeeze the metatarsophalangeal joints between the first and fifth metatarsals to check for tenderness.
- Palpate individual interphalangeal joints.
- Repeat for the other foot/ankle.

Move

- Evaluate active movements of the ankles.
- Ask the patient to point the toes towards the ceiling (dorsiflexion).
- Ask the patient to point the toes towards the floor (plantar flexion).
- Fix the patient's heel with one hand and ask the patient to turn the sole in towards the mid-line (inversion).
- Fix the patient's heel with one hand and ask the patient to turn the sole away from the mid-line (eversion).
- Evaluate active movements of the toes.
- Ask the patient to curl the toes (toe flexion).
- Ask the patient to straighten the toes (toe extension).

- Ask the patient to fan the toes (toe abduction).
- Ask the patient to close the toes together (toe eversion).
- Evaluate passive movements of the ankles and toes.
- Repeat all the above by actively providing the movements.

Special test
Simmonds' test

- Where indicated, perform this test to identify a rupture of the Achilles' tendon (Kesson & Atkins, 2005).
- Ask the patient to kneel on a chair, with the feet hanging over the edge.
- Squeeze the gastrocnemius (calf muscle) gently (Figure 7.10); normally, the foot will plantar flex, but no plantar flexion will occur if the Achilles' tendon is ruptured.

EXAMINATION OF THE WRIST AND HAND

- Expose both hands and forearms.
- Compare both sides.

Look

- Look at the wrists and the dorsal and palmar aspects of the hands for scars, deformity, abnormal hand posture, swelling and muscle wasting.
- Look at the nails for abnormalities, such as pitting, onycholysis (separation of the nail from its bed) and discoloration (Talley & O'Connor, 2006).

Feel

- Check whether there is any tenderness before proceeding.
- Palpate the wrist joint, metacarpophalangeal joint, proximal interphalangeal joint and distal phalangeal joint of the fingers and interphalangeal joint of the thumb.

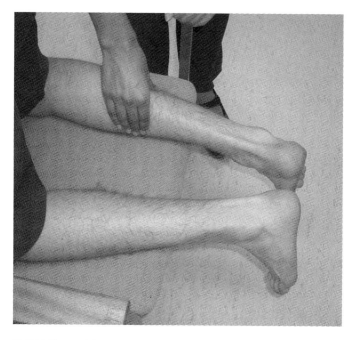

Fig 7.10 Simmonds' test to identify a rupture of the Achilles' tendon: ask the patient to kneel on a chair, with the feet hanging over the edge, and gently squeeze the gastrocnemius (calf muscle)

- During palpation of each joint, note any tenderness, temperature, swelling and bony abnormality.
- Feel the palm for evidence of thickening of the palmar fascia as seen in Dupuytren's contracture (Figure 7.11).

Move

- Evaluate active movements of the wrist, noting any limitation, discomfort and presence of crepitus.

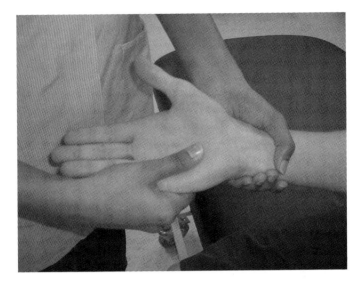

Fig 7.11 Palpation of the palm

- Ask the patient to adopt a prayer position with the hands (dorsiflexion or extension); the normal range of movement is up to 75°.
- Ask the patient to adopt an inverse prayer position with the hands (flexion); the normal range of movement is up to 75°.
- Ask the patient to move the wrist towards the thumb (radial deviation); the normal range of movement is up to 20°.
- Ask the patient to move the wrist towards the little finger (ulnar deviation); the normal range of movement is up to 20°.
- Evaluate active movements of the fingers, noting any limitation, discomfort and presence of crepitus.

- Ask the patient to make a fist (flexion) and open it out (extension).
- Ask the patient to spread the fingers apart (abduction).
- Ask the patient to close the fingers back together (adduction).
- Evaluate active movements of the thumb, noting any limitation, discomfort and presence of crepitus.
- Ask the patient to curl in the thumb (flexion) and straighten it out (extension).
- With the palm facing the ceiling, ask the patient to lift the thumb up, pointing it towards the ceiling (abduction), and back down (adduction).
- Ask the patient to touch the tip of each individual finger using the tip of the thumb of the same hand (opposition).
- Evaluate passive movements of the wrist and hand.
- Repeat all the above movements by moving the patient's wrists, fingers and thumbs; note any limitation, discomfort and presence of crepitus.

Special tests
Trigger finger

- Ask the patient to make a fist and release it quickly; triggering is present if the finger (or thumb) is locked or caught as it is extended (thickening of the tendon sheath may prevent straightening of the fingers).

Carpal tunnel syndrome
The exact mechanism of this condition is uncertain, but compression of the median nerve in the carpal tunnel is involved (Kesson & Atkins, 2005). If carpal tunnel syndrome is suspected, the following tests can be conducted.

1 *Tinel's test*:
   ○ Tap over the carpal tunnel on the flexor aspect of the wrist (Figure 7.12); the test is positive when the symptoms of carpal tunnel syndrome (pins and needles in the radial three and a half fingers) are reproduced.

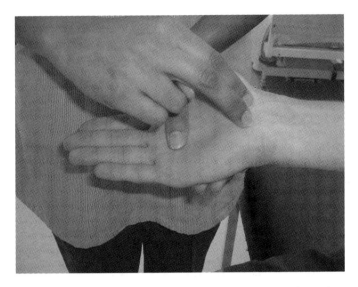

Fig 7.12 Tinel's test: tap over the carpal tunnel on the flexor aspect of the wrist

2   *Phalen's test*:
   ○ Hold the patient's hands in the inverse prayer position (i.e. wrist flexion) for 60 s (Figure 7.13). The test is positive when the symptoms of carpal tunnel syndrome (pins and needles in the radial three and a half fingers) are reproduced.

EXAMINATION OF THE SPINE

• Expose the cervical, thoracic and lumbar spines.

Look

• Inspect for scars, deformity, swelling and abnormal curvatures, such as kyphosis (exaggerated curvature of the thoracic spine causing a rounded upper back), lordosis (exaggerated curvature of the lumbar spine causing a sway back) and scoliosis (spine curving to the side).

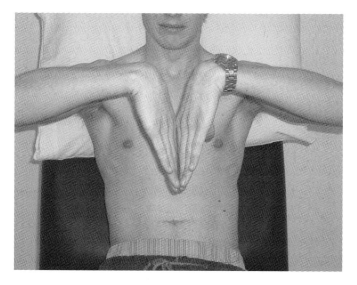

Fig 7.13 Phalen's test: hold the patient's hands in the inverse prayer position (i.e. wrist flexion) for 60 s

Feel

- Using the thumb, feel the spinous processes along the spine starting from the base of the skull to check for abnormal gaps and tenderness (Figure 7.14).
- Palpate the paraspinal muscles next to the spine for spasm and tenderness.

Move

- Evaluate active movements of the cervical spine, noting any limitation and discomfort.
- Ask the patient to look down at the toes (flexion).
- Ask the patient to look up at the ceiling (extension).
- Ask the patient to look over each shoulder in turn (lateral rotation).

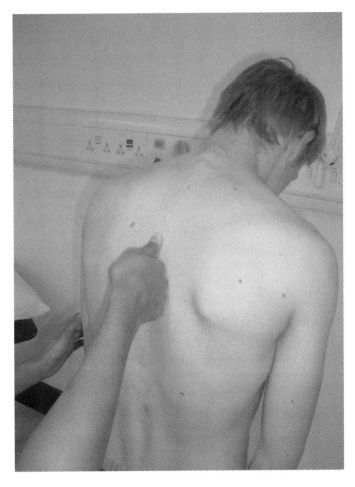

Fig 7.14 Palpation of the spinal processes

- Ask the patient to put each ear onto the shoulder in turn (lateral flexion); to ensure that the patient does not shrug the shoulders, fix them when assessing this movement.
- Evaluate active movements of the thoracic and lumbar spine, noting any limitation and discomfort.

- Ask the patient to touch the toes without bending the knees (flexion).
- Ask the patient to lean backwards as far as possible (extension).
- Secure the pelvis and ask the patient to turn at the waist in turn (lateral rotation).
- Ask the patient to slide the hand down the side of each leg in turn (lateral flexion).
- Evaluate passive movements of the cervical, thoracic and lumbar spines.
- Repeat all the above movements, actively moving the patient's cervical, thoracic and lumbar spines, noting any limitation and discomfort.

Special tests

Schober's test

This test is used to assess spinal flexion (Douglas *et al.*, 2005).

- Ask the patient to stand with the back exposed.
- Locate and draw a line at the level of the posterior superior iliac spine (dimples of Venus); then mark two points at 10 cm above and 5 cm below this line. Place a tape measure between the two points (Figure 7.15).
- Ask the patient to bend forwards as far as possible without bending the knees. The two points should separate by at least 5 cm on flexion in healthy individuals; any value less than this may indicate pathology affecting the lumbar spine, e.g. ankylosing spondylitis.

Straight leg-raising test

This test is used to assess sciatic nerve root compression (Kesson & Atkins, 2005).

- Lie the patient supine.
- Lift the patient's leg upwards without bending the knee (Figure 7.16); normally, raising a straight leg to 90° in the supine patient should be painless. In the presence of sciatic nerve root

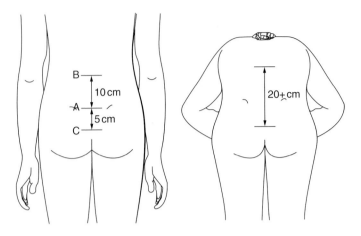

Fig 7.15 Schober's test to assess spinal flexion

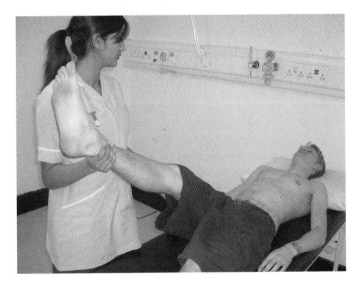

Fig 7.16 Straight leg-raising test to assess sciatic nerve root compression

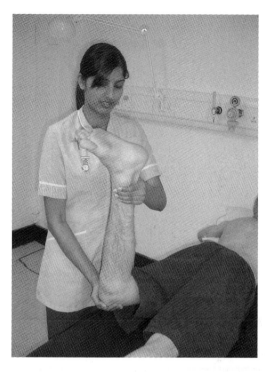

Fig 7.17 Lifting the patient's leg upwards with an extended knee to check for the presence of femoral nerve root compression

compression, the patient will feel a radiating pain from the lower back to below the knee.

Femoral stretch test (reverse leg-raising test)

This test is used to assess femoral nerve root compression (Kesson & Atkins, 2005).

- Ask the patient to lie prone.
- Lift the patient's leg upwards with an extended knee (Figure 7.17); in the presence of femoral nerve root compression, the patient will feel pain down the front of the leg to the knee.

CONCLUSION

The diagnosis of musculoskeletal or rheumatological problems can be made following detailed history taking, sound physical examination and, where indicated, appropriate investigations, e.g. X-rays. Examination of the musculoskeletal system involves the look (inspection), feel (palpation) and move (active and passive) approach. In some situations, special tests can be performed on certain joints to elicit further clinical features to aid in the diagnosis. This chapter has provided an overview to the principles of examination of the musculoskeletal system.

REFERENCES

Abrahams PH, Craven JL, Lumley JSP (2005) *Illustrated Clinical Anatomy*. Hodder Arnold, London.

Cox NLT, Roper TA (2005) *Clinical Skills: Oxford Core Text*. Oxford University Press, Oxford.

Douglas G, Nicol F, Robertson C (2005) *MacLeod's Clinical Examination*, 11th edn. Elsevier, Edinburgh.

Ford M, Hennessey I, Japp A (2005) *Introduction to Clinical Examination*. Elsevier, Oxford.

Gleadle J (2004) *History and Examination at a Glance*. Blackwell Publishing, Oxford.

Kesson M, Atkins E (2005) *Orthopaedic Medicine: a Practical Approach*, 2nd edn. Elsevier, Edinburgh.

Moore KL, Dalley AF (2006) *Clinically Oriented Anatomy*, 5th edn. Lippincott Williams & Wilkins, Philadelphia, PA.

Talley NJ, O'Connor S (2006) *Clinical Examination: a Systematic Guide to Physical Diagnosis*, 5th edn. Elsevier, Edinburgh.

Assessment of the Critically Ill Patient

8

INTRODUCTION

The approach to clinical examination described in this book is not appropriate in the critically ill patient. In this possibly life-threatening situation, the patient must be assessed quickly following the recommended ABCDE approach (Resuscitation Council UK, 2006), and any adverse physiological signs, e.g. tachycardia, tachypnoea or hypotension, should be identified quickly and treated effectively; cardiopulmonary arrest may then be prevented (Adam & Osborne, 2005).

The aim of this chapter is to provide an understanding of the assessment of the critically ill patient.

LEARNING OUTCOMES

At the end of this chapter, the reader will be able to:

❏ Outline the ABCDE approach.
❏ Outline the initial approach to the patient.
❏ Describe the assessment of the airway.
❏ Describe the assessment of breathing.
❏ Outline the assessment of circulation.
❏ Describe the assessment of disability.
❏ Outline the importance of exposure.

ABCDE APPROACH

The ABCDE approach can be used for the assessment and treatment of a critically ill patient. The guiding principles are as follows:

This chapter is based on the chapter 'Assessment of the Critically Ill Patient', which first appeared in *Monitoring the Critically Ill Patient* by Jevon & Ewens (2007). It has been revised and updated.

- Follow a systematic approach based on *A*irway, *B*reathing, *C*irculation, *D*isability and *E*xposure (ABCDE) to assess and treat the critically ill patient.
- Undertake a complete initial assessment; reassess regularly. Always treat life-threatening problems first, before proceeding to the next part of the assessment.
- Always evaluate the effects of treatment and/or other interventions.
- Recognize the circumstances in which additional help is required; request it early and utilize all members of the multi-disciplinary team. This will enable the assessment, instigation of monitoring, intravenous access, etc. to be undertaken simultaneously.
- Ensure effective communication. Call for help early.

(Resuscitation Council UK, 2006)

The ABCDE approach can be used by all healthcare practitioners, irrespective of their training, experience and expertise in clinical assessment and treatment: clinical skills and knowledge will determine what aspects of the assessment are undertaken (Resuscitation Council UK, 2006).

'The underlying aim of the initial interventions should be seen as a 'holding measure' to keep the patient alive, and produces some clinical improvement, in order that definitive treatment may be initiated' (Resuscitation Council UK, 2006).

INITIAL APPROACH TO THE PATIENT
Ensure that it is safe to approach the patient: check the environment and remove any hazards. Measures should also be taken to minimize the risk of cross-infection (Box 8.1).

Ask the patient a simple question
Ask the patient a simple question, e.g. 'how are you?'. The patient's response or lack of response can provide valuable information. A normal verbal response implies that the patient has a patent airway, is breathing and has cerebral perfusion; if the patient can only speak in short sentences, extreme respiratory

Box 8.1 Minimizing the risk of cross-infection

Measures to minimize the risk of cross-infection should be taken. It is estimated that 5000 deaths per year are directly associated with hospital-acquired infection (HAI) and, in 15 000 deaths per year, it is a contributory factor (Plowman *et al.*, 1997). The principal route of HAI is via the hands (Casewell & Phillips, 1977; Elliott, 1992; Bursey *et al.*, 2001). Effective hand hygiene is recognized as the most effective intervention to prevent cross-infection [Larsen, 1999; Bissett 2003; National Institute for Clinical Excellence (NICE), 2003], and the simplest (Voss & Widmer, 1997).

NICE (2003) issued guidance governing the principles of good practice relating to handwashing:

- Hands must be decontaminated immediately before every episode of direct patient contact or care after any activity or contact that could potentially have resulted in the hands becoming contaminated.
- Hands that are visibly soiled or potentially grossly contaminated with dirt or organic material must be washed with liquid soap and water.
- Hands must be decontaminated, preferably with an alcohol-based handrub, unless hands are visibly soiled, between caring for different patients and between different care activities for the same patient.
- Before regular hand decontamination begins, all wrist and, ideally, hand jewellery should be removed. Cuts and abrasions must be covered with waterproof dressings. Fingernails should be kept short, clean and free from nail polish.
- An effective handwashing technique involves three stages: preparation, washing and rinsing, and drying. Preparation requires the wetting of hands under tepid running water before applying liquid soap or an antimicrobial preparation. The handwash solution must come into contact with all surfaces of the hand. The hands must be rubbed together vigorously for a minimum of 10–15 s, paying particular attention to the tips of the fingers, the thumbs and the areas between the fingers. Hands should be rinsed thoroughly before drying with good-quality paper towels.

Continued

- When decontaminating hands using an alcohol handrub, hands should be free from dirt and organic material. The handrub solution must come into contact with all surfaces of the hand. The hands must be rubbed together, paying particular attention to the tips of the fingers, the thumbs and the areas between the fingers, until the solution has evaporated and the hands are dry.
- An emollient handcream should be applied regularly to protect the skin from the drying effects of regular hand decontamination. If a particular soap, antimicrobial handwash or alcohol product causes skin irritation, an occupational health team should be consulted.

For hygienic hand disinfection, an antiseptic solution will need to be used, e.g. chlorhexidine (Bursey *et al.*, 2001). This category of handwashing should be used during an infection outbreak, prior to aseptic techniques and when the hands have been contaminated with body fluids (Kerr, 1998). It is also recommended to use hygienic hand disinfection in particularly vulnerable patients, e.g. those who are immunodepressed, those in intensive treatment units and newborn babies (Horton & Parker, 1997).

Universal precautions to blood and bodily fluids

Blood is the single most important source of transmission of human immunodeficiency virus (HIV) and hepatitis B virus (Jevon, 2002). Universal precautions should apply to blood, semen, vaginal secretions and cerebrospinal, synovial, pleural, peritoneal, pericardial and amniotic fluids, and any body fluid containing visible blood (Centers for Disease Control, 1988). Disposable gloves should be donned.

Sharps

Particular care should be taken with sharps as both HIV and hepatitis B virus have been contracted by healthcare workers following needle-stick injuries (Marcus, 1988).

distress may be present; failure to respond is a clear indication of serious illness (Resuscitation Council UK, 2006). An inappropriate response or no response indicates that the patient may be critically ill.

NB: if the patient is unconscious, summon help from colleagues immediately.

General appearance of the patient

Note the general appearance of the patient (comfortable or distressed, content or concerned) and the colour of the patient.

Monitoring of vital signs

The monitoring of vital signs, e.g. pulse oximetry, electrocardiogram (ECG) and continuous non-invasive blood pressure, should be performed as soon as it is safe to do so (Resuscitation Council UK, 2006).

ASSESSMENT OF THE AIRWAY

If the patient is talking, there is a patent airway. In complete airway obstruction, there are no breath sounds at the mouth or nose. In partial obstruction, air entry is diminished and often noisy. The familiar look, listen and feel approach can detect whether the airway is obstructed.

Look

Look for the signs of airway obstruction. Airway obstruction leads to paradoxical chest and abdominal movements ('see-saw' respirations) and the use of the accessory muscles of respiration. Central cyanosis is a late sign of airway obstruction.

Listen

Listen for signs of airway obstruction. Certain noises will assist in localizing the level of the obstruction (Smith, 2003):

- *Gurgling*: fluid in the mouth or upper airway.
- *Snoring*: tongue partially obstructing the pharynx.
- *Crowing*: laryngeal spasm.
- *Inspiratory stridor*: 'croaking respirations' indicating partial upper airway obstruction, e.g. foreign body, laryngeal oedema.

- *Expiratory wheeze*: noisy musical sound caused by turbulent flow of air through narrowed bronchi and bronchioles, more pronounced on expiration; causes include asthma and chronic obstructive airway disorder.

Feel

Feel for the signs of airway obstruction. Place your face or hand in front of the patient's mouth to determine whether there is movement of air.

Causes of airway obstruction

The causes of airway obstruction include:

- *Tongue*: this is the most common cause of airway obstruction in a semiconscious or unconscious patient; relaxation of the muscles supporting the tongue can result in it falling back and blocking the pharynx.
- *Vomit, blood and secretions*.
- *Foreign body*.
- *Tissue swelling*: causes include anaphylaxis, trauma and infection.
- *Laryngeal oedema*: causes include burns, inflammation or allergy occurring at the level of the larynx.
- *Laryngeal spasm*: causes include foreign body, airway stimulation or secretions/blood in the airway.
- *Tracheobronchial obstruction*: causes include aspiration of gastric contents, secretions, pulmonary oedema fluid or bronchospasm.

(Sources: Smith, 2003; Gwinnutt, 2006)

Treatment of airway obstruction

Treat airway obstruction as a medical emergency and obtain expert help immediately; untreated, airway obstruction leads to a lowered P_aO_2 and risks hypoxic damage to the brain, kidneys and heart, cardiac arrest and even death (Resuscitation Council UK, 2006).

Once airway obstruction has been identified, treat appropriately. Simple methods, e.g. suction, lateral position or insertion of an oropharyngeal airway, are often effective. Administer oxygen as appropriate.

The assessment of the patient's airway is described in more detail in Chapter 4.

ASSESSMENT OF BREATHING

The familiar look, listen and feel approach can be used to assess breathing to detect signs of respiratory distress or inadequate ventilation (Smith, 2003).

Look

Look for the general signs of respiratory distress: tachypnoea, sweating, central cyanosis, use of the accessory muscles of respiration and abdominal breathing (Resuscitation Council UK, 2006).

Calculate the respiratory rate over 1 min. The respiratory rate is the most useful sign that breathing is compromised (Smith, 2003). The normal respiratory rate in adults is approximately 12–20 breaths/min (Resuscitation Council UK, 2006). Tachypnoea is usually one of the first indicators of respiratory distress (Smith, 2003). If the respiratory rate is high or increasing, this may indicate that the patient is ill and may suddenly deteriorate (Resuscitation Council UK, 2006).

Bradypnoea is an ominous sign, and possible causes include drugs (opiates), fatigue, hypothermia, head injury and central nervous system depression. Sudden bradypnoea in a patient with respiratory distress may quickly be followed by respiratory arrest.

Assess the depth of breathing. Ascertain whether the chest movement is equal on both sides. Unilateral movement of the chest suggests unilateral disease, e.g. pneumothorax, pneumonia or pleural effusion (Smith, 2003). Kussmaul's breathing (air hunger) is characterized by deep rapid respirations as a result of stimulation of the respiratory centre by metabolic acidosis, e.g. in ketoacidosis and chronic renal failure.

Assess the pattern (rhythm) of breathing. A Cheyne–Stokes breathing pattern (periods of apnoea alternating with periods of hyperpnoea) can be associated with brain stem ischaemia, cerebral injury and severe left ventricular failure (altered carbon dioxide sensitivity of the respiratory centre) (Ford *et al.*, 2005).

Note the presence of any chest deformity, as this could increase the risk of deterioration of the patient's ability to breathe normally (Resuscitation Council UK, 2006). If the patient has a chest drain, check that it is patent and functioning effectively. The presence of abdominal distension could limit diaphragmatic movement, thereby exacerbating respiratory distress.

Document the inspired oxygen concentration (%) being administered to the patient and the oxygen saturation (S_aO_2) reading of the pulse oximeter (normally 97–100%). NB: the pulse oximeter does not detect hypercapnia and, if the patient is receiving oxygen therapy, S_aO_2 may be normal in the presence of a very high P_aCO_2 (Resuscitation Council UK, 2006).

Listen

Listen to the patient's breath sounds a short distance from the face. Normal breathing is quiet. Rattling airway noises indicate the presence of airway secretions, usually either because the patient is unable to cough sufficiently or is unable to take a deep inspiratory breath (Smith, 2003). Stridor or wheeze suggests partial, but significant, airway obstruction (see above).

If able, auscultate the chest: the depth of breathing and the equality of breath sounds on both sides of the chest should be evaluated. Any additional sounds, e.g. crackles, wheeze or pleural rubs, should be noted. Bronchial breathing indicates lung consolidation; absent or reduced sounds suggest a pneumothorax or pleural fluid (Smith, 2003).

Feel

Perform chest percussion. The causes of different percussion notes are as follows:

- *Resonant*: air-filled lung.
- *Dull*: liver, spleen, heart, lung consolidation/collapse.
- *Stony dull*: pleural effusion/thickening.
- *Hyper-resonant*: pneumothorax, emphysema.
- *Tympanitic*: gas-filled viscus.

(Source: Ford *et al.*, 2005)

Check the position of the trachea. Place the tip of the index finger into the suprasternal notch; let it slip either side of the trachea and determine whether it fits more easily on one side of the trachea (Ford *et al.*, 2005). Deviation of the trachea to one side indicates a mediastinal shift (e.g. pneumothorax, lung fibrosis or pleural fluid).

Palpate the chest wall to detect surgical emphysema or crepitus (suggesting a pneumothorax *until* proven otherwise) (Smith, 2003).

Efficacy of breathing, work of breathing and adequacy of ventilation

- *Efficacy of breathing* can be assessed by air entry, chest movement, pulse oximetry, arterial blood gas analysis and capnography.
- *Work of breathing* can be assessed by respiratory rate and accessory muscle use, e.g. neck and abdominal muscles.
- *Adequacy of ventilation* can be assessed by heart rate, skin colour and mental status.

Causes of compromised breathing

The causes of compromised breathing include:

- Respiratory illness, e.g. asthma, chronic obstructive pulmonary disease, pneumonia.
- Lung pathology, e.g. pneumothorax.
- Pulmonary embolism.
- Pulmonary oedema.
- Central nervous system depression.
- Drug-induced respiratory depression.

Treatment of compromised breathing

If the patient's breathing is compromised, position appropriately (usually upright), administer oxygen and, if possible, treat the underlying cause. Expert help should be summoned. Assisted ventilation may be required. During the initial assessment of breathing, it is essential to diagnose and treat effectively immediately life-threatening conditions, e.g. acute severe asthma, pulmonary oedema, tension pneumothorax and massive haemothorax (Resuscitation Council UK, 2006).

The assessment of the patient's breathing is discussed in more detail in Chapter 4.

ASSESSMENT OF CIRCULATION

In most medical and surgical emergencies, if shock is present, treat for hypovolaemic shock until proven otherwise (Smith, 2003). Administer intravenous fluid to all patients who have tachycardia and cool peripheries, unless the cause of circulatory shock is obviously cardiac (cardiogenic shock) (Resuscitation Council UK, 2006). In surgical patients, haemorrhage should be rapidly excluded. The familiar look, listen and feel approach can be used for the assessment of circulation.

Look

Look at the colour of the hands and fingers. Signs of cardiovascular compromise include cool and pale peripheries.

Measure the capillary refill time. A prolonged capillary refill time (>2 s) may indicate poor peripheral perfusion, although other factors, e.g. cool ambient temperature, poor lighting and old age, may also be responsible (Resuscitation Council UK, 2006).

Look for other signs of a poor cardiac output, e.g. reduced conscious level and, if the patient has a urinary catheter, oliguria (urine volume, <0.5 ml/kg/h) (Smith, 2003).

Examine the patient for signs of external haemorrhage from wounds or drains or evidence of internal haemorrhage. Concealed blood loss can be significant, even if the drains are empty (Smith, 2003).

Listen

Measure the patient's blood pressure. A low systolic blood pressure suggests shock. However, even in shock, the blood pressure can still be normal, as compensatory mechanisms increase peripheral resistance in response to reduced cardiac output (Smith, 2003). A low diastolic blood pressure suggests arterial vasodilatation (e.g. anaphylaxis or sepsis). A narrowed pulse pressure, i.e. the difference between the systolic and diastolic pressures (normal pulse pressure is 35–45 mmHg), suggests arterial vasoconstriction (e.g. cardiogenic shock or hypovolaemia) (Resuscitation Council UK, 2006).

Auscultate the heart. Although abnormalities of the heart valves can be detected, auscultation of the heart is rarely helpful in the initial assessment (Smith, 2003).

Feel

Assess the skin temperature of the patient's limbs to determine whether they are warm or cool, the latter suggesting poor peripheral perfusion.

Palpate the peripheral and central pulses. Assess for the presence, rate, quality, regularity and equality (Smith, 2003). A thready pulse suggests a poor cardiac output, and a bounding pulse may indicate sepsis (Resuscitation Council UK, 2006).

Assess the state of the veins: if hypovolaemia is present, the veins could be underfilled or collapsed (Smith, 2003).

Causes of circulatory compromise

The causes of circulatory problems include:

- Acute coronary syndromes.
- Cardiac arrhythmias.
- Shock, e.g. hypovolaemia, septic and anaphylactic shock.
- Heart failure.
- Pulmonary embolism.

Treatment of circulatory compromise

The specific treatment required for circulatory compromise will depend on the cause; fluid replacement, haemorrhage control and restoration of tissue perfusion will usually be necessary (Resuscitation Council UK, 2006).

The immediate treatment for a patient with an acute coronary syndrome includes oxygen, aspirin 300 mg, sublingual glyceryl trinitrate and morphine (diamorphine); reperfusion therapy will need to be considered (Resuscitation Council UK, 2006). If shock is present, a large-bore cannula (12–14 gauge) should be inserted and an intravenous fluid challenge will usually be required.

The assessment of the patient's circulation is discussed in more detail in Chapter 3.

ASSESSMENT OF DISABILITY

The assessment of disability involves an evaluation of central nervous system function. Undertake a rapid assessment of the patient's level of consciousness using the AVPU method (Table 6.1, p. 126) (the Glasgow Coma Scale can also be used). Causes of an altered conscious level include hypoxia, hypercapnia, cerebral hypoperfusion, the recent administration of sedatives/analgesic medications and hypoglycaemia (Resuscitation Council UK, 2006). Therefore:

- Review ABC to exclude hypoxaemia and hypotension. Check the patient's drug chart for reversible drug-induced causes of an altered conscious level.
- Undertake bedside glucose measurement to exclude hypoglycaemia.
- Examine the pupils (size, equality and reaction to light).

(Resuscitation Council UK, 2006)

Causes of an altered conscious level

The causes of an altered conscious level include:

- Severe hypoxia.
- Poor cerebral perfusion.
- Drugs, e.g. sedatives, opiates.
- Cerebral pathology.
- Hypercapnia.
- Hypoglycaemia.
- Alcohol.

Treatment of an altered conscious level

The first priority is to assess ABC: exclude or treat hypoxia and hypotension (Resuscitation Council UK, 2006). If a drug-induced altered conscious level is suspected and the effects are reversible, administer an antidote, e.g. naloxone for opiate toxicity. Administer glucose if the patient is hypoglycaemic.

The assessment of the patient's conscious level is discussed in more detail in Chapter 6.

EXPOSURE

Full exposure of the patient may be necessary in order to undertake a thorough examination and to ensure that important details are not overlooked (Smith, 2003). In particular, the examination should concentrate on the part of the body which is most likely to be contributing to the patient's ill status, e.g. in suspected anaphylaxis, examine the skin for urticaria. The patient's dignity should be respected and heat loss minimized.

In addition:

- Undertake a full clinical history.
- Review the patient's case notes, observations' chart and medications' chart.
- Study the recorded vital signs: trends are more significant that one-off recordings.
- Ensure that prescribed medications are being administered.
- Review the results of laboratory, ECG and radiological investigations.

- Consider the level of care required by the patient (e.g. ward, high-dependency unit, intensive care unit).
- Record in the patient's case notes the details of assessment, treatment and response to treatment.

(Source: Resuscitation Council UK, 2006)

CONCLUSION

The recognition and effective treatment of critically ill patients are paramount. The ABCDE approach of assessing the critically ill patient has been described and the importance of calling for help early has been emphasized.

REFERENCES

Adam S, Osborne S (2005) *Critical Care Nursing Science and Practice*, 2nd edn. Oxford University Press, Oxford.

Bissett L (2003) Interpretation of terms used to describe handwashing activities. *Br J Nursing* **12**(9): 536–542.

Bursey S, Hardy C, Gregson R (2001) Handwashing. *Prof Nurse* **16**(10): 1417–1419.

Casewell M, Phillips I (1977) Hands as route of transmission for *Klebsiella* species. *Br Med J* **2**: 1315–1317.

Centers for Disease Control (1988) Update: universal precautions for prevention of transmission of immunodeficiency virus, hepatitis virus and other blood-borne pathogens in healthcare settings. *Morb Mortal Wkly Rep* **37**: 377–388.

Elliott P (1992) Hand washing: a process of judgement and effective decision making. *Prof Nurse* **2**: 292–296.

Ford M, Hennessey I, Japp A (2005) *Introduction to Clinical Examination*. Elsevier, Oxford.

Gwinnutt C (2006) *Clinical Anaesthesia*, 2nd edn. Blackwell Publishing, Oxford.

Horton R, Parker L (1997) *Informed Infection Control Practice*. Churchill Livingstone, London.

Jevon P (2002) *Advanced Cardiac Life Support: A Practical Guide*. Butterworth Heinemann, Oxford.

Jevon P, Ewens B (2007) *Monitoring the Critically Ill Patient*, 2nd edn. Blackwell Publishing, Oxford.

Kerr J (1998) Handwashing. *Nurs Stand* **12**(51): 35–42.

Larsen E (1999) Skin hygiene and infection prevention: more of the same or different approaches? *Clin Infect Dis* **29**: 1287–1294.

Marcus R (1988) CDC Cooperative Needlestick Surveillance Group. Surveillance of health care workers exposed to blood from patients infected with the human immunodeficiency virus. *N Engl J Med* **319**: 1118–1123.

National Institute for Clinical Excellence (NICE) (2003) *Infection Control: Prevention of Healthcare-Associated Infection in Primary and Community Care*. NICE, London.

Plowman R, Graves N, Roberts J (1997) *Hospital Acquired Infection*. Office of Health Economics, London.

Resuscitation Council UK (2006) *Advanced Life Support*, 5th edn. Resuscitation Council UK, London.

Smith G (2003) *ALERT Acute Life-Threatening Events Recognition and Treatment*, 2nd edn. University of Portsmouth, Portsmouth.

Voss A, Widmer A (1997) No time for hand-washing? Handwashing vs alcohol rubs: can we afford 100% compliance? *Infect Control Hosp Epidemiol* **18**: 205–208.

Record Keeping

9

INTRODUCTION

'Record keeping is an integral part of nursing and midwifery' [Nursing and Midwifery Council (NMC), 2008]. 'It is a tool of professional practice and one that should help the care process. It is not separate from this process and it is not an optional extra to be fitted in if circumstances allow' (NMC, 2005). When taking a history and undertaking a clinical examination, the nurse must ensure that accurate and good records are kept.

The aim of this chapter is to provide an understanding of good record keeping.

LEARNING OUTCOMES

At the end of this chapter, the reader will be able to:

❏ Discuss the importance of good record keeping.
❏ List the common deficiencies in record keeping.
❏ Discuss the principles of good record keeping.
❏ Outline the legal issues associated with record keeping.

IMPORTANCE OF GOOD RECORD KEEPING

Good record keeping will help to protect the welfare of both the patient and the nurse by promoting:

• High standards of clinical care.
• Continuity of care.

This chapter is based on the chapter 'Record Keeping', which first appeared in *Monitoring the Critically Ill Patient* by Jevon & Ewens (2007). It has been revised and updated.

- Better communication and dissemination of information between members of the interprofessional healthcare team.
- The ability to detect problems, such as changes in the patient's condition, at an early stage.
- An accurate account of treatment and care planning and delivery.

The quality of record keeping is also a reflection on the standard of nursing practice: good record keeping is an indication that the practitioner is professional and skilled, whereas poor record keeping often highlights wider problems with the individual's practice (NMC, 2005).

COMMON DEFICIENCIES IN RECORD KEEPING

Nearly every report published by the Health Service Commissioner (Health Service Ombudsman) following a complaint identifies examples of poor record keeping that have either hampered the care that the patient has received or have made it difficult for healthcare professionals to defend their practice (Dimond, 2005).

Commonly encountered deficiencies in record keeping include:

- Absence of clarity.
- Failure to record the action taken when a problem has been identified.
- Missing information.
- Spelling mistakes.
- Inaccurate records.

(Dimond, 2005)

PRINCIPLES OF GOOD RECORD KEEPING

There are a number of factors that underpin good record keeping. The patient's records should:

- Be factual, consistent and accurate.
- Be updated as soon as possible after any recordable event.

- Provide current information on the care and condition of the patient.
- Be documented clearly and in such a way that the text cannot be erased.
- Be consecutive and accurately dated, timed and signed (including a printed signature).
- Have any alterations and additions dated, timed and signed; all original entries should be clearly legible.
- Not include abbreviations, jargon, meaningless phrases, irrelevant speculation and offensive subjective statements.
- Still be legible if photocopied.
- Identify any problems and, most importantly, the action taken to rectify them.

It is important to record all aspects of the clinical examination of the patient.

Best practice – record keeping
Records must be:

- Factual.
- Legible.
- Clear.
- Concise.
- Accurate.
- Signed.
- Timed.
- Dated.

(Drew *et al.*, 2000)

NMC guidance on record keeping
The NMC (2008) stresses the importance of clear and accurate records. A nurse or midwife must:

- Keep clear and accurate records of any discussions undertaken, any assessments made, any treatment and medicines given, and the effectiveness of these treatments.

- Complete the records as soon as possible after an event has occurred.
- Not tamper with original records in any way.
- Ensure that any entries made in an individual's paper records are clearly and legibly signed, dated and timed.
- Ensure that any entries made in an individual's electronic records are clearly attributable to the nurse or midwife making the entry.
- Ensure that all records are kept confidentially and securely.

LEGAL ISSUES ASSOCIATED WITH RECORD KEEPING

The patient's records are occasionally required as evidence before a court of law, by the Health Service Commissioner or in order to investigate a complaint at a local level. Sometimes they may be requested by the NMC's Fitness to Practice committees when investigating complaints related to misconduct. Care plans, diaries and anything that makes reference to the patient's care may be required as evidence (NMC, 2005).

What constitutes a legal document is often a cause for concern. Any document requested by the court becomes a legal document (Dimond, 1994), e.g. nursing records, medical records, X-rays, laboratory reports, observation charts; in fact, any document which may be relevant to the case.

If any of the documents are missing, the writer of the records may be cross-examined as to the circumstances of their disappearance (Dimond, 1994). 'Medical records are not proof of the truth of the facts stated in them but the maker of the records may be called to give evidence as to the truth as to what is contained in them' (Dimond, 1994).

The approach to record keeping adopted by courts of law tends to be that if it is not recorded, it has not been undertaken (NMC, 2005). Professional judgement is required when deciding what is relevant and what needs to be recorded, particularly if the patient's clinical condition is apparently unchanging and no record has been made of the care that has been delivered.

A registered nurse has both a professional and a legal duty of care. Consequently, when keeping records, it is important to be able to demonstrate that:

- A comprehensive nursing assessment of the patient has been undertaken, including care that has been planned and provided.
- Relevant information is included, together with any measures that have been taken in response to changes in the patient's condition.
- The duty of care owed to the patient has been honoured and no acts or omissions have compromised the patient's safety.
- Arrangements have been made for the ongoing care of the patient.

The registered nurse is also accountable for any delegation of record keeping to members of the multiprofessional team who are not registered practitioners. For example, if record keeping is delegated to a pre-registration student nurse or a healthcare assistant, competence to perform the task must be ensured and adequate supervision provided. All such entries must be countersigned.

The Access to Health Records Act 1990 gives patients the right of access to their manually maintained health records which were made after 1 November 1991. The Data Protection Act 1998 gives patients the right to access their computer-held records. The Freedom of Information Act 2000 grants the rights to anyone to all information that is not covered by the Data Protection Act 1998 (NMC, 2005).

Sometimes it is necessary to withhold information, if it could affect the physical or mental well-being of the patient, or if it would breach another patient's confidentiality (NMC, 2005). If the decision to withhold information is made, justification for doing so must be clearly recorded in the patient's notes.

CONCLUSION

This chapter has provided an overview to good record keeping. The importance of good record keeping has been discussed. The common deficiencies in record keeping have been highlighted and the principles of good record keeping have been described. The legal issues associated with record keeping have been outlined.

REFERENCES

Dimond B (1994) *Legal Aspects in Midwifery.* Books for Midwives Press, Altrincham, Cheshire.

Dimond B (2005) Exploring common deficiencies that occur in record keeping *Br J Nursing* **14**(10): 568–570.

Drew D, Jevon P, Raby M (2000) *Resuscitation of the Newborn.* Butterworth Heinemann, Oxford.

Jevon P, Ewens B (2007) *Monitoring the Critically Ill Patient*, 2nd edn. Blackwell Publishing, Oxford.

Nursing and Midwifery Council (NMC) (2005) *Guidelines for Records and Record Keeping*. NMC, London.

Nursing and Midwifery Council (NMC) (2008) *The Code: Standards of Conduct, Performance and Ethics for Nurses and Midwives*. NMC, London.

Index